Cybertraps for Expecting Moms & Dads

By Frederick S. Lane

PUBLISHED BY

Frederick S. Lane

Cybertraps for Expecting Moms & Dads
Original Copyright 2016 Frederick S. Lane
Version 1.00

Cover Design by Colin Gliech
On LinkedIn: http://www.linkedin.com/in/colingliech

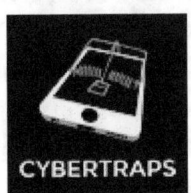

Introduction

The idea for this book arose out a series of conversations I had with my former upstairs neighbor, Tami Mnoian, not long after the birth of her daughter in early 2015. Tami knew about my research and work in the area of cybersafety, and mentioned that she and some other new mothers had a number of questions about pregnancy-related technology and privacy issues. She thought that a book summarizing and discussing those issues would be helpful. So here it is — not quite as quickly as I planned, but still timely.

My initial plan was to write a short e-book focusing solely on the privacy issues involving women who are actually pregnant, as well as their spouses, partners, family members, *etc.*, *etc.*. As I began exploring this topic in more depth, however, it quickly became apparent that technology is having a warp field effect on virtually every aspect of human reproduction, from the first hints of emoji-laced courtship to the moment a newly-sentient human being is handed his or her first digital device.

As someone who researches, writes, and lectures about emerging technologies and privacy (among other topics), I was already aware of the enormous interest that retailers and manufacturers have in families who are expecting a baby. Pregnant women are one of the most valuable target demographics in the advertising business (just ahead of pre-mid-life crisis men), since they are a sure bet to spend hundreds, if not thousands of dollars on pregnancy and newborn supplies.

After researching this topic, however, I concluded that it's only a small but useful stretch to expand the definition of "expecting moms and dads" to include pretty much anyone of child-bearing years, or frankly, anyone who hopes one day to become a grandparent. That's not to say that everyone in that demographic will have children. In fact, as we'll see, there's considerable concern about the falling birthrate among millennials. A couple's decision to have a child or not is a conversation well beyond the scope of this book. But one of the goals of *Cybertraps for Expecting Moms & Dads* is to remind those who might someday procreate, or who are under seemingly endless pressure from parents to do so, that there are technological issues that they should consider long before they start posting photos of their pregnancy test stick or first sonogram on Facebook or Instagram.

In contemporary society, it is important to acknowledge that the phrase "expecting mom and dad" is no longer synonymous, to the extent it ever fully was, with "husband and wife." I intend the phrase to encompass married and unmarried heterosexual couples, married and unmarried gay couples, single parents, and the myriad other variations on family structure that exist in our society. To reflect that intent, I have avoided the use of "husband," "wife," and "spouse," and have used the term "partner" to encompass all of the people who collaborate intimately or otherwise in the conception, birthing, and rearing of a child. My sincere wish is for every mother to have the partner or partners she needs throughout pregnancy and beyond.

Above all, the purpose of this book is not to present vast quantities of detailed research data; I'll leave that to formally-trained social scientists and Ph.D. candidates. Instead, my intent to provide a thoughtful and hopefully entertaining overview of some of the more interesting issues that possible, soon-to-be, and even new parents should consider. My hope is that this book will spur reflection and conversation among potential parents about the numerous effects that technology is having on the seemingly straightforward process of creating a new human being. In many ways, we can thank technology for making us better informed about procreation and pregnancy than ever before; more often than not, however, we are unaware that the identical technology is informing Web site owners, advertisers, retailers, and even the government about the details of this most intimate and fascinating of human events.

Overview of the Book

So what exactly is a "cybertrap"? I define the term as follows: "an unintended or unexpected consequence resulting from the use and/or misuse of a digital device, a social media platform, or any other form of electronic communication." As will become evident, some of the issues that I discuss in this book predate the digital era; what brings those issues into the category of "cybertraps" is the remarkable speed with which those issues now arise, the potential for the global spread of collected information, and the unforeseen threats arising out of the increasingly powerful mining of data, much of it user-generated.

This book is divided into three parts. The first section deals with pre-conception cybertraps, from courtship to fertilization. The second section covers cybertraps that arise during pregnancy itself. The third section takes a look at some of cybertraps that can arise during the birth of a child and during the first bleary, sleep-deprived days and weeks of new parenthood.

Section One: The Cybertraps of Conception

Disconcertingly, there is a possibility that our use of mobile devices in particular may damage the quality of our reproductive cells years before we actually try to conceive. In **Chapter One**, I take a look at the debate over the impact of mobile technology on human fertility.

It is much more difficult, although not impossible, for someone to conceive if he or she has been severely injured or has died in an accident. In **Chapter Two**, I discuss the ways in which our obsession with mobile devices is heightening our risk of serious physical injury and even death.

In **Chapter Three**, I look at the myriad ways in which technology in general and mobile devices in particular are changing dating and courtship. In **Chapter Four**, I examine the possible impact that mobile apps like Grindr and Tinder are having on the incidence of sexually transmitted infections (STIs) [I.1] and pregnancy rates in general.

In the normal course of events, intercourse is a necessary predicate to pregnancy. **Chapter Five** raises the questions of whether our numerous digital devices are either preventing or interfering with the emotional and physical intimacy that facilitates procreation.

"There's an App for That (Even If You Don't Know It)." As digital devices and mobile apps play a bigger and bigger role in our everyday lives, those tools often know much more about our physical health and mental state than we do. **Chapter Six** explores the ways in which digital devices and services might know that you are pregnant before you do.

Section Two: Your Little Bundle of Data

Chapter Seven begins the discussion of cybertraps during pregnancy, beginning with social media posts of pregnancy tests and the etiquette of contemporary pregnancy announcements.

In **Chapter Eight**, I revisit some of the physical harm that can result from the use of mobile devices, but this time with a focus on the impact on the developing fetus.

One of the main areas of concentration of my work is personal privacy. **Chapter Nine** explores the tremendous economic value of your personal data when pregnant and the privacy issues that inevitably arise.

Chapter Ten brings the discussion back to social media, through a discussion of some of the issues you and your partner might want to consider during the course of your pregnancy. The primary question, as always, is how much do you want to share and with whom. Underlying that question should be the realization that once you share, it is virtually impossible to maintain control over the spread and use of that information.

Section Three: The Cybertraps of Birthing and Infancy

As your newborn gets ready to make an appearance, you will want to think about who will be present in the delivery room to meet him or her, and how the new arrival should be announced. **Chapter Eleven** reviews some of the pitfalls that can arise.

Choosing a name for your baby can be an exciting process. It can be an opportunity to merge two family identities, reaffirm traditions, or acknowledge some meaningful aspect of the parents' relationship. Thanks to technology and the realities of online identification, as **Chapter Twelve** illustrates, it can also be frustrating and complicated.

New parents, particularly those in the millennial generation, will see an endless wave of "smart" parenting products marketed to them. **Chapter Thirteen** reviews some of the options and highlights potential concerns.

With the arrival of a newborn, parents are immediately confronted with serious decisions about how their own use of technology will affect their child. **Chapter Fourteen** illustrates the need for every parent of a newborn to think carefully about the example they are setting.

In **Chapter Fifteen**, I look at the issue of self-determination. Parents need to balance between their desire to share kid photos with relatives and friends, and the right of any child to shape his or her own identity. It is a task made much more difficult when there are hundreds or thousands of photos of him or her on social media.

Chapter Sixteen presents increasingly powerful medical evidence that child use of digital devices should be delayed as long as possible. Are mobile devices replacing the television as our *de facto* babysitter? If so, what are the possible consequences for kids themselves and society as a whole?

Any couple that is expecting or is planning to do so should take the time to write out a digital technology plan to discuss assumptions, expectations, and values. **Appendix A** contains a list of topics and guiding questions to facilitate that discussion.

A Brief Word Regarding the References in the Text

I have organized notes and references by chapter; they can be found towards the end of book in the section labeled "Endnotes." The material referenced in the endnotes is drawn from my research files, which have been compiled over the past twenty years, as well as ongoing research that I have done specifically for this project. In many cases, I have copies of articles which may have been moved from the original electronic location, or which may be from sources that no longer exist. Every effort has been made to provide thorough and accurate citations, but inevitably, it may not be possible to access some of these articles directly. If anyone is attempting to locate a cited article that cannot be found online, please feel free to contact me through the contact form on my Web site.

The Internet Is Changeable

At various points in this book, I have referred to various devices, products, apps, software, privacy policies, and terms of service. Each of those items was online and viewable at the time this book was published but there is no guarantee, nor do I offer one, that any of the items is available and unchanged at the time you are reading this. Even if one or more changes has occurred in the specific items I cite, the lessons I've drawn from these examples are still relevant. Undoubtedly, similar examples can easily be found.

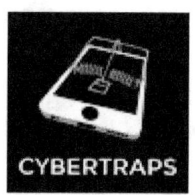

Section One
The Cybertraps of Conception

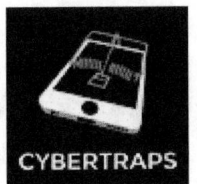

Chapter One

Mobile Technology and Human Fertility: A Heated Debate

Few people today would argue that technology has been anything other than a blessing to expecting moms and dads. *In vitro* fertilization has helped thousands of infertile couples start a family; for the last fifty years, electronic fetal monitors have provided physicians with critical information about the health of the fetus during delivery; sonograms provide a precious first glimpse of new life and valuable data throughout pregnancy; wireless monitors now give mothers more mobility during labor; the list goes on and on. [1.1]

But for all of the benefits bestowed by technological innovation, the unfortunate reality is that those innovations also present us with unexpected challenges and unintended consequences. Portable music players, for instance, have enabled us to take our own personal music libraries with us wherever we go but those same devices are blamed for a rise in hearing loss among even casual users. [1.2] Many of the most popular personal tech devices on the market today have been linked to claims of environmental damage or the use of child labor in overseas factories. [1.3] And no one really foresaw that teens would use cell phones to bully other teens or take nude photos of themselves. We can now add to that list the increasingly pressing question of whether our obsession with mobile devices, particularly smartphones, makes it less likely that we can or will have children.

Our Favorite Technology

Without question, no recently-invented device has infused itself into our daily lives as thoroughly as the cell phone. Although mobile phones were first developed in the early 1970s, it wasn't until the 1990s that consumer use of the technology really took off. According to statistics compiled by CITA — The Wireless Association, a mobile industry trade group, there were just 3.5 million cell phone subscribers in the United States at the beginning of 1990. By the end of the decade, there were roughly 86 million subscribers, or nearly 30 times as many. [1.4] Today, the number of mobile phone users in the United States alone has risen to approximately 260 million people [1.5] and of those, more than 190 million are using a smartphone. [1.6]

It's not terribly surprising that smartphones have become so incredibly popular. A single device that can fit in our pocket now allows us to keep in touch with family and friends, take photographs, shoot high-quality video, read books, play music, navigate through the world, look up an endless amount of information, and stay up to date on the latest news. Given the tremendous versatility of these devices, it's also no great shock that people are spending an enormous amount of time with their smartphones each day. In a 2013 study conducted by the research firm IDC for Facebook, for instance, 63% of smartphone owners reported carrying their device or keeping it near them all but one hour of their waking day. Nearly 80% put the within-arms-reach estimate at all but two hours. When respondents were asked how this made them feel, the overwhelming response was "connected." That makes sense, given the fact that the primary use of the devices — more than two hours each day — is to communicate with others in some fashion — text, email, social media, and occasionally (just 16% of the time), by voice. [1.7]

Predictably, cell phone use by millennials is particularly intense. IDC found that among 18-24 year olds, 9 out of 10 reach for their phone with 15 minutes of first waking up. [1.8] More recently, the Pew Research Center found that 83% percent of 18-29 year olds report turning their phones off "rarely" or "never." [1.9]

Given the fact that an estimated 5 billion people around the world today are cell phone subscribers, and given the steady increases in the amount of time these devices are used each day in close proximity to our bodies, scientists are naturally eager to determine whether cell phone technology poses any health risk to humans. If so, the potential costs, both personal and global, are tremendous. It didn't take long for researchers to start sounding alarms that the design and operation of cell phones might be causing unanticipated health issues for users. To better understand this intense debate, it is helpful to have a basic idea of how cell phones actually work.

Cell Phone Technology

All cell phones use radio-frequency (RF) waves to transmit voice and data from the handset to the nearest cell tower or WiFi receiver. RF waves are a form of electromagnetic energy with frequencies that fall between

FM radio on the low end and microwaves on the high end. This type of energy is not generally considered to be harmful; it is typically described as *non-ionizing* radiation, *i.e.,* a type of radiation not powerful enough (we are fairly sure) to cause health problems such as cancer by penetrating our cells and altering our DNA. By contrast, more powerful types of radiation, such as X-rays, gamma rays, and ultraviolet light, have well-documented and highly negative effects on human cells, and are collectively referred to as *ionizing* radiation. [1.10]

During the course of a phone conversation, the antenna in your cell phone generates RF waves to transmit your voice to the nearest cell tower. Those RF waves move out from your phone in an omni-directional fashion, which means that some RF waves are inevitably traveling through your head and being absorbed by your body. That is one reason, for instance, that some health professionals strongly recommend the use of ear buds. For each cell phone or smartphone on the market, scientists calculate what is known as the *specific absorption rate* for the device, *i.e.,* the number of watts absorbed per kilogram of human tissue (W/kg). The Federal Communications Commission, which regulates the use of cell phones in the United States, has ruled that a cell phone may not have a specific absorption rate in excess of 1.6 W/kg; the European Union has a slightly higher threshold of 2.0 W/kg. [1.11]

As the American Cancer Society puts it, RF radiation is just strong enough to "to get atoms in a molecule a little bit excited and to cause them to vibrate," but not strong enough to either alter the atoms themselves or break apart the molecules in our cells. However, quantity matters; with sufficient amounts of RF radiation, it is possible to generate heat in various substances by causing the water molecules in those substances to vibrate so rapidly that they heat up their surroundings. That is precisely how a microwave works to cook or reheat beverages and food. The energy generated by the average cell phone handset causes minimal heating of the tissue near the handset, but scientists are still conducting research to determine the biological effects of repeated heating of the same tissue or long-term exposure of human tissue to low-level but persistent increases in heat. [1.12]

The amount of power used by your handset to generate the necessary RF waves is generally modest but not constant; the level ebbs and flows over the course of the day. There are a number of different factors that come into play. For instance, different models of phones use different levels of RF energy and have different SAR values; among other things, you might want to research and compare SAR values when you are shopping for a new phone. If you are using your phone in a congested area where lots of other conversations are taking place (an airport, for instance, or Grand Central Station), the handset will need to use more power to transmit. Similarly, the power required to carry your communication increases the farther you are from the nearest cell tower, or if there is some sort of barrier between you and the cell tower. You may have noticed, for instance, that your battery drains more quickly when the phone is attempting to connect in a remote area or from the inside of a building.

The amount of RF energy generated by your phone drops significantly when you are not using it to talk to someone or surf the Web, but it does not stop altogether. Even when your phone is in "standby" mode, *i.e.*, simply waiting for a call, it is still communicating with the nearest cell phone tower to let your cellular service provider know where to find you so that calls can be routed to your handset. Those ongoing pings between handsets and cell towers, incidentally, offer a remarkably detailed record of your movements over the course of a day; it is information that can be of great interest and use to law enforcement during a criminal investigation. The only way to eliminate RF waves altogether is to shut your phone down completely and leave it off.

What particularly concerns medical researchers is the fact that cell phones and smartphones spend the bulk of each day in one of two locations: Either pressed up against your head during a call, or resting near your groin, since cell phones are most commonly carried in a front pants pocket or a purse. That means that the RF waves generated by these devices routinely pass through two particularly sensitive parts of our bodies: our brains and our reproductive organs.

Are Cell Phones Making Us Less Fertile?

The debate over whether cell phones cause cancer or other significant health problems is long-running, contentious, and generally beyond the scope of this book. The Web is peppered with sites that offer grim assessments of the gruesome illnesses cause by cell phones, electromagnetic radiation, cell phone towers, *etc.* However, the general scientific consensus so far seems to be that cell phones do not cause brain tumors or other forms of cancer in our heads.

One of the earlier studies of the effects of RF radiation, published in 1999, was largely dismissive of any negative effects:

The epidemiological evidence for an association between RF radiation and cancer is found to be weak and inconsistent, the laboratory studies generally do not suggest that cell phone RF radiation has genotoxic or epigenetic activity, and a cell phone RF radiation-cancer connection is found to be physically implausible. Overall, the existing evidence for a causal relationship between RF radiation from cell phones and cancer is found to be weak to nonexistent. [1.13]

Much more recently, an extensive study of data from a 29-year period in Australia found that despite a sharp increase in cell phone usage across the continent, approaching 90% of Australians, there has been no corresponding increase in the incidence of brain cancer. [1.14]

While we can all breathe easier that our beloved smartphones are probably not going to turn our brains into Swiss cheese, that does not mean that smartphones are completely off the hook when it comes to deleterious health effects. The data regarding the effects of RF radiation on human fertility — particularly for men — are far more equivocal and worrisome.

Impact of RF Radiation on Female Fertility

One would think, given the profound importance of the female reproductive system to the perpetuation of the human species, that any potential threat to the functioning of that system would be thoroughly and intensively examined. And generally speaking, that does happen; the *Guardian* reported last year that U.S. specialists in female fertility outnumber those specializing in men by five to one. [1.15] Remarkably enough, however, when it comes to cell phones, it appears that the opposite is true.

In an article dated April 2, 2014, *Parenting* asked an important question: "Do Cell Phones Harm Female Fertility?" The answer was chilling: "As scary as it may be to consider that such things could affect female fertility," Victoria Georgoff wrote, "the fact is we just don't know yet." She put the blame for the lack of answers on the unprecedented levels of device use, the brief period of time during which these devices have been used, and the fact that unlike men, the female reproductive organs are in the center of the body rather than dangling outside. [1.16]

We'll get to the dangling bits in a minute, but Georgoff's initial explanations are simply not adequate excuses. If anything, the unprecedented levels of device usage by women should be a powerful incentive for much more research in this area. Moreover, significant numbers of women have been using cell phones for at least twenty years, and some for much longer than that. While it can take years for meaningful health data to emerge from the background noise and statistical clutter generated by millions of individual human decisions, it does seem like more of an effort should be made to figure out if cell phones are posing a threat to the ability of women to bear children.

Another area that deserves careful study is the possible connection between cell phones and breast cancer. A study published in 2013 chronicled four cases of women, ages 21 to 39, who developed tumors in their breasts in the same location in which they carried a cell phone tucked into their bra for hours every day over a period of years. All four had no other known breast cancer risks. As the authors put it, "[t]hese cases raise awareness to the lack of safety data of prolonged direct contact with cellular phones." [1.17]

Obviously, while breast cancer does not have a direct impact on a woman's ability to conceive or bear a child, some of the side-effects to cancer treatment can interfere with both.

Impact of RF Radiation on Male Fertility

Make of it what you will, but there is no lack of research or scientific literature about the potential effects of cell phone RF radiation on the male reproductive system. Some readers may attribute the focus on men to mere sexism; given the apparent disparity in research levels in this area, it's hard not to have some sympathy for that point of view. Clearly, more balanced levels of research are needed.

There may be many reasons for the disparity in research expenditures, but here is perhaps the most significant: There is growing evidence that men around the world have been experiencing a significant and deeply troubling decline in fertility over the last several decades. There are three key components to male fertility: the number of sperm a man produces, the health of the sperm (the extent to which it is free from defect or deformity), and sperm motility (the ability of sperm to wiggle their way from the back of the vagina through the uterus and on to the fallopian tubes). If any one of those components is substandard, a man's fertility is compromised; the more damage to each aspect of sperm health, the less likely it is that the man can father a child.

In 1992, a paper published in *British Medical Journal* concluded that over a fifty year period, the concentration of sperm in collected samples had fallen by half, from 113 million sperm per milliliter to 66 million. [1.18] Similarly, in 2012, Israeli sperm banks reported that over a ten-year period, the number of donors meeting their fertility standards dropped from 1 in 10 to 1 in 100, due to issues with both quantity of sperm and motility. [1.19] Most recently, a team of French researchers at the Institut de Veille Sanitaire, St Maurice, conducted a study of 26,000 men from 1989 to 2005; their examination of sperm samples showed that the number of sperm in the samples had dropped by over a third during that period. The researchers also found that on average, the collected sperm samples showed a similar decline in the percentage of healthy or normally formed sperm. [1.20]

As with the sudden and sharp rise in bumble bee mortality, it's one thing to identify a problem in male sperm health and another thing to explain it. A variety of different causes have been postulated, ranging from the overheating effects of tightie-whities to excessive levels of lead in the environment to the potent petrochemical cocktail that surrounds us every day. One of the leading suspects in that latter medical drama, according to researchers in Copenhagen, is a class of chemicals known as pthlates, which are used to make plastics more flexible and less prone to breakage. [1.21]

For more than a decade, some researchers have speculated that cell phone technology may be exacerbating the problem. In 2004, researchers at the University of Szeged, Hungary presented findings that suggested that RF radiation from a cell phone could cut the number of healthy sperm in a man by a third. [1.22] Similar findings were reported in 2005 by the University of Newcastle in the United Kingdom, in 2008 in the journal *Fertility & Sterility*, in 2011 by researchers at Queen's University in Canada, in 2014 by researchers at the University of Exeter in the U.K., and most recently by a team at Haifa University in Israel. [1.23]

While these studies all concluded that there appeared to be some connection between cell phone use and damage to sperm, there is less consensus as to how exactly mobile devices are contributing to the problem. Some researchers believe that sperm, which are particularly delicate cells, can be harmed by electromagnetic radiation in general and RF radiation in particular; others pointed to the heating effects of RF radiation or the heat generated by cell phones during their normal operation. According to medical experts, testicles hang outside the male body because the optimum temperature for sperm production is 1 to 2° C below the typical body core temperature of 37° C. Men who are trying to conceive with their partner are routinely advised to avoid hot tubs and heated car seats [1.24], and now some physicians are recommending that men keep cell phones away from their reproductive factories as well.

It's important to keep in mind that this is a topic that is still hotly debated. As one scientist sarcastically wrote following the latest doom-and-gloom study last winter, "No, cell phones are not 'cooking men's sperm.'" [1.25] Even if sperm quantity and quality is declining worldwide, there are undoubtedly multiple causes and cell phones may only be a tiny part of the problem. The only thing that we know for certain is that we are running a massive experiment on ourselves and we won't know the outcome for years.

In the interim, if you are worried, then consult a fertility specialist, think about keeping your phone as far away from your body as is practical, and perhaps give some thought to purchasing some anti-radiation boxer shorts on Amazon — just $90 a pair but hey, what price fertility?

A Brief Warning for Men about Laptops

As I discuss later in the book (*see* Chapter 8), laptop computers are chiefly an issue for pregnant women to consider, both in terms of the heat they produce and the radiation that they emit. However, given the sensitivity of sperm cells to increases in heat, laptops do appear may pose a threat to male fertility. In a study led by Dr. Yefim Sheynkin, a urologist at the State University of New York at Stony Brook, researchers found that when men use a laptop as designed — on their laps — the temperature of their scrotum quickly rises to levels that are unhealthy for sperm. Remarkably, research shows that damage to sperm can occur when testicular temperatures rise as little as 1° Celsius. Dr. Sheynkin conceded that no one had specifically researched the impact of laptop use on male fertility, but noted that he and his researchers had measured testicular temperature increases by laptop users as high as 2.5° Celsius. [1.26]

The only foolproof solution, researchers said, was to put laptop computers on a desk. While lap pads do keep laptop computers cooler, they don't do much to prevent overheating of the testicles, particular when men keep their legs together. Actually, the much-reviled "manspreading" may have a biological value; by keeping the legs apart while using a laptop computer, a man can slow the heating process. However, researchers said, dangerous levels of heat still occurred within as little as 30 minutes. [1.27]

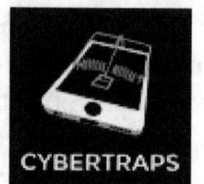

CYBERTRAPS

Chapter Two

Death from Digital Distraction and Other Missed Conceptions

The bulk of this book is devoted to cataloging and considering the myriad risks to personal privacy posed by digital devices and social media during pregnancy, from the instant of conception through the first hazy, blurry days of parenthood. Without question, those are the most pervasive cybertraps that expecting moms and dads will face. But logically enough, there's no point in discussing those privacy risks and other cybertraps if there's no pregnancy in the first place. Over the next several chapters, we will examine the ways in which our use of cell phones and smartphones may be interfering with our ability to reproduce.

The most serious impediment to human reproduction, of course, is death; as general rule, once you die, your days of splashing around in the human gene pool are over. [2.1] Back in April 1973, when Motorola employee Martin Cooper made the first cellular phone call from midtown Manhattan to Bell Labs in New Jersey, it is doubtful that he or anyone else really imagined that mobile phones would ever pose any kind of threat to human life. But over the course of the last half century or so, cell phones have become a contributing factor in a startlingly large number of deaths each year.

Are You a 'Smombie'?

By far, the greatest number of fatalities stem from the toxic combination of cell phones and automobiles. In 2010, researchers from the University of North Texas Health Science Center published one of the first studies attempting to quantify the human cost. Fernando Wilson and Jim Stimpson estimated that between 2001 and 2007, "[d]rivers distracted by talking or texting on cell phones killed an estimated 16,000 people[.]" [2.2] More recently, the National Safety Council estimated that more than a quarter of all driving accidents in 2013 were caused by the use of cell phones. That represented a total of more than 1.5 *million* collisions. It was also the third year in a row that the number of cell phone-related accidents had risen. [2.3]

A variety of different test results help explain why cell phones make driving so much more dangerous. University of Utah researchers used a driving simulator in 2006 to compare the reaction times of drivers talking on a cell phone with inebriated drivers. They concluded: "The data presented in this article … indicate that when driving conditions and time on task are controlled for, the impairments associated with using a cell phone while driving can be as profound as those associated with driving with a blood alcohol level at 0.08% [the legal limit of intoxication while driving]." [2.4]

Similarly, in the summer of 2009, *Car and Driver* tested driver reaction times to a simulated red light while reading an email, sending a text message, and driving drunk (the tests were conducted, fortunately, on an empty airport runway in Michigan). The results were startling; both test drivers took longer to respond to the red light while using their phone compared to driving drunk. In fact, the magazine's 37-year-old test subject took twice as long to hit the brakes while reading a text as he did with nearly half of a fifth of vodka in him. [2.5]

> In our test, neither subject had any idea that using his phone would slow down his reaction time so much. Like most folks, they think they're pretty good drivers. Our results prove otherwise, at both city and highway speeds. The key element to driving safely is keeping your eyes and your mind on the road. Text messaging distracts any driver from that primary task. [2.6]

But sometimes, it's not the driver who is distracted but the pedestrian. In 2015, the U.S. government reported the first increase in pedestrian deaths in decades. An Ohio State University study found that the 3.5 percent of pedestrian deaths in 2010 occurred while the pedestrian was using his or her cell phone. By comparison, in 2004, that figure was just 1 percent. Researchers also point out that pedestrians using their cell phones are less likely to observe basic road safety rules, such as looking both ways or obeying traffic lights, and take longer to actually cross from one side of the street to the other. [2.7]

The phenomenon is known as "distracted walking," and not surprisingly, teenage pedestrians are at greatest risk. Four in ten teens report that they have been hit or nearly hit by a car, motorcycle or bike, and cell phone distraction is a factor in a significant percentage of those cases. [2.8]

According to Dr. Dietrich Jehle, a professor of emergency medicine at the University of Buffalo, "distracted walking" is actually more dangerous per mile traveled than distracted driving. People using their cell phones while walking, he said, are hampered by three different types of distraction: "manual, in which they are doing something else; visual, where they see something else; and cognitive, in which their mind is somewhere else." [2.9]

Thanks to YouTube, we have access to a nearly endless supply of "America's Funniest Cell Phone Videos" showing people bumping into or falling off things — walls, fountains, subway platforms, brown bears — while distracted by their phones. The videos may be amusing, but the humor obscures the very real and serious physical injuries that can result from these accidents, including bruises, abrasions, cuts, fractures, concussions, and even death. [2.10] In fact, the problem has become so acute that in 2015, the National Safety Council for the first time "included statistics on cell phone distracted walking." Among other things, the NSC reported that between 2000 and 2011, distracted walking resulted in over 11,000 injuries; 54% of the accidents involved people under 40 and 68% of those injured were female. [2.11]

Given the human toll from distracted walking, cities around the world are trying a variety of different methods to minimize the risks. Nearly a decade ago, for instance, London officials wrapped lampposts on Brick Lane in East London with the same type of padding used to wrap football or rugby goal posts; a quick Google Image search will show that while public safety may have been improved, the visual appeal of Brick Lane was badly damaged. In 2004, ABC News aired a segment on "texting while walking" that showed some distracted walking YouTube clips and noted that the town of Fort Lee, NJ was planning to start fining people who paid more attention to their phones than their surroundings. [2.12] Other municipal solutions for what the Germans refer to as "smombies" (a remarkably inelegant portmanteau of "smartphone" and "zombie.") include: traffic lights embedded in the ground at dangerous intersections (Augsburg and Cologne); traffic beacons that send a heads-up alert to phones on which the "Watch Out!" app has been installed (Munich); talking buses to alert pedestrians (Portland, Seattle and Cleveland); and a dedicated sidewalk cell phone lane (Chongqing). [2.13]

The take-away from all of this is fairly simple: you should avoid looking at your phone while walking and simply enjoy your surroundings — you never know what you might see. But if you simply can't bring yourself to stop texting or using social media as you walk, then you might want to consider one or more of the safety apps that are beginning to appear in the iTunes or Google Play stores. In addition to the previously mentioned "Watch Out!," apps like "SafeNote" or "Type n Walk" use your phone's camera to show you what is ahead of you as you type on the screen; it's as if you are typing your message on a window. Of course, for such apps to be most effective, you need to get into the habit of typing your messages while holding your phone pointing forward as opposed to pointing down. If you can bring to do so, however, you may find that the health of your neck will improve as well.

On the other hand, it may be that the "transparent camera" approach actually doesn't offer much of a safety advantage. On July 6, 2016, Nintendo released an "augmented reality" game called "Pokémon Go," which requires smartphone players to physically move around while searching for different types of Pokémon (fictional creatures that players attempt to capture). When a Pokémon is found, the game can display it on a generated map or by using the phone's camera to make it appear that the creature is located in the real world. Already, several Pokémon Go players have injured themselves by focusing on the game and not on their surroundings. [2.14]

Other researchers are working on apps that will alert you to possible dangers by using artificial intelligence to evaluate your surroundings by analyzing images from your camera in real time to identify known obstacles such as cars, curbs or lampposts. Others think similar results can be achieved by using your phone's microphone to listen for potential dangers, like the squealing brakes of the car that's about to hit you. [2.3] It remains to be seen whether smartphones can process that type of data as quickly as each of us could if we simply paid attention to where we are going.

Fatal Narcissism

As further proof that there is nothing new under the sun, consider the ancient Greek legend of Narcissus, a beautiful young man who saw his reflection in a forest pool and fell in love with it. Unable to reach or touch the beautiful youth he saw in the pool, Narcissus pined away and eventually died. In other variations of the story, he tries to kiss his reflection, falls into the pool, and drowns. The name of that pool, if it ever had one, is lost to the mists of time, but we know its modern day equivalents: Facebook, Instagram, and Snapchat.

Narcissus unwittingly lent his name to the psychiatric condition we know today as "narcissism," which is defined as "too much interest in and admiration for your own physical appearance and/or your own abilities." [2.16] In extreme cases, narcissism can develop into a psychiatric disorder called Narcissistic Personality Disorder (NPD), which is marked by "an inflated sense of importance, a deep need for admiration and a lack of empathy for others." [2.17]

Interest in narcissism has been fueled by the perception among many psychiatrists and sociologists that our society is growing steadily more narcissistic. A long-term study, for instance, has shown that the percentage of college students who demonstrate narcissistic personality traits has doubled since the 1980s. [2.18] If you are curious to see how high you score, a version of the Narcissistic Personality Inventory is available online. A parallel study has shown a corresponding decline in empathy, for reasons that I will discuss later in this book. Both trends are disturbing and raise difficult questions about the kind of society in which we want to live. Among other things, more narcissistic individuals place greater value on various types of extrinsic validation — money, image, fame, social media "likes," *etc.* — than they do on community and collaboration. [2.19]

Nothing better reflects the rise of narcissism in our society than our obsession with the "selfie," the ubiquitous arms-length or mirror self-portraits that flood social media. To be fair, this is not an entirely new phenomenon: People have been taking photos of themselves for close to 200 years, and painting them long before that. The first known photographic "self-portrait," for instance, is an image that American photograph Robert Cornelius created of himself in the fall of 1839, just a few months after the daguerreotype process was publicized in the United States. [2.20] Other technologies, like the Polaroid camera in the 1970s and 1980s, and the digital camera in the 1990s and 2000s, have also been widely used to take self-portraits.

Today's "selfie" phenomenon, however, is different in both scale and scope, thanks to the technological *ménage à trois* of the Internet, cameraphones, and social media. In 2000, electronics firm Sharp first began marketing cell phones with a built-in camera. That innovation sped up both the creation and the distribution of selfies by making it possible for users to take a photo and immediately send it electronically to family, friends, or the entire Web. [2.21] The concept of putting a camera in a phone has proven staggeringly popular: by 2014, there were 4 billion cameras in use around the world. Of those, 3.56 billion were part of a cameraphone. One expert estimated that for the first time, humans took over one *trillion* photos in a single year. [2.22]

Even more remarkable is the percentage of those photos that are selfies; and here, millennials, I'm looking squarely at you and your social media feeds. At the end of 2015, one organization estimated that 93 million selfies are taken every single day. 95% of teenagers have taken a selfie of themselves, and 30% of the photos taken by teens overall are selfies. [2.23] The selfie craze grew so rapidly and embedded itself so deeply into our cultural DNA that the *Oxford English Dictionary* pronounced "selfie" as its "Word of the Year" in 2013. The *OED* traced the origin of the term to a 2002 forum comment by an Australian named Nathan Hope on the Australian Broadcasting Company Web site, when he uploaded a photo of stitches on his lip:

> Um, drunk at a mates 21st, I tripped ofer [sic] and landed lip first (with front teeth coming a very close second) on a set of steps. I had a hole about 1cm long right through my bottom lip. And sorry about the focus, it was a selfie. [2.24]

There is some irony in the fact that the *OED* cited that particular photo in its origin story, since Hope's photo was far more honest and self-deprecating than the vast majority of the billions of selfies that have been taken in the fourteen years since. There is legitimate concern about the myriad ways that the selfie phenomenon reinforces negative body images for millennials and in particular, for young women. At the extreme end of the spectrum, many who are obsessed with selfies suffer from a psychological condition known as Body Dysmorphic Disorder (BDD), in which sufferers obsess about one or more perceived flaws in their appearance and spend enormous amounts of time examining themselves in mirrors and/or trying to take an absolutely perfect selfie. [2.25] As we'll see, this is an issue that arises with varying degrees of severity for women during and after pregnancy.

There are a number of reasons that expecting moms and dads, and even prospective grandparents, should be concerned about the rise of narcissism and selfie culture.

First, BDD is a serious mental illness that can interfere with various aspects of a person's emotional and physical health, including the ability to conceive, pregnancy, and parenthood. In its most severe manifestations, it can lead to suicidal ideation or even suicide attempts.

Second, narcissists, and especially those suffering from narcissistic personality disorder, are neither the best prospective partners nor the most optimal parents. There are dozens of different books about narcissists in print right now, many of which directly focus on the impact of narcissism on family relationships:

- Freeing Yourself from Narcissist in Your Life;
- Will I Ever Be Good Enough? Healing the Daughters of Narcissistic Mothers; and
- Divorcing a Narcissist: Rebuilding After The Storm.

Long before you decide to have a child with someone, it is worth exploring whether these issues might possibly present a problem for you and your child. Professor Jean Twenge, author of the The Narcissism Epidemic: Living in the Age of Entitlement, actually made her future husband take the Narcissistic Personality Inventory on their fourth date. Fortunately for him, his score apparently was not disqualifying. [2.26]

Third, if you are a narcissistic/obsessive taker and poster of selfies, that behavior will affect your child in several negative ways. I'll discuss this in more detail in other sections of the book, but suffice it to say that it will it interfere with the bond between you and your newborn, it will set a bad example for your child, it will distract you from parenting over the course of their childhood, and it will increase the risk that you will effectively define your child's online identity before he or she has a chance to do so.

Fourth and most dramatically, the combination of youthful risk-taking and the inherent narcissism of selfies can be fatal. In January 2016, a data analysis site called Priceonomics reviewed reports of 49 selfie-related deaths dating back to 2014. They found that the average age of the decedents was 21, 75% of the victims were male, and remarkably, nearly half the incidents occurred in India. A plurality of deaths, roughly one-third, occurred because the deceased fell from a high height — typically off a cliff or the edge of a building. The second largest cause of death was drowning (14 cases), followed by trains (8 cases) and then gunshots (4 cases). [2.27]

One fairly typical victim of selfie-inflicted wounds was a 17-year-old Russian named Andrey Retrovsky. His Instagram feed, **@drewsssik**, which is still viewable online, contains several photos of him and selfies he took on the rooftops of his home town, Vologda. As part of his effort to feed his rapidly growing audience of nearly 5,000 followers, he planned a stunt photo in which he would pretend to be falling off the edge of a 9-

story building. But as he positioned himself over the side of the building, the rope he was holding snapped. Retrovsky fell to the ground and died two hours later in a nearby hospital. [2.28] Ironically, just two months earlier, the Russian government had issued a public service guide for the taking of safe selfies. Among other things, the government warned that people should not take selfies with guns, on railway lines (a problem in the U.S. as well), or on the roof of tall buildings. [2.29] There is no way to know if Retrovsky ever saw his government's warnings but if he did, they clearly made little impression.

The social-media-fueled hunt for the most dramatic Instagram or Facebook photo is driving people to the brink, quite literally. In Brazil, tourists are flocking to Pedra da Gavea, a 2,769 ft-high rock on the outskirts of Rio de Janeiro. The cliff offers dramatic views of the city far below, but the images of people standing, sitting, or even dangling from the cliff face are stomach-churning. [2.30] Similarly, hundreds of tourists each month are making a 10-hour round-trip hike in Norway so that they can take photos on or from a dramatic rock formation called Trolltunga (literally, "troll's tongue") that sticks out from a cliff face more than 2,000 feet above Lake Ringedalsvatnet. [2.31] Local guides say that the formation only became widely popular following the advent of social media. One reporter described the scene:

> It's really terrifying watching people walk out and get their photos taken. Many don't realise that the walk to the rock is a really tough route, taking up to 10 hours up and down, and are taken aback at just how difficult a climb it is. I met two Americans who were incredulous about the lack of toilets en route and were calling for a road right to the top. Others were annoyed at the lack of 3G, delaying their Facebook posting. Once you reach the top, climbers queued for their chance to take a photo on the spectacular plateau. Despite the wind, and the narrow ledge, groups of people were jumping in the air, sitting with their legs dangling over the edge and, of course - taking selfies. [2.32]

Trolltunga claimed its first victim just three weeks before Retrovsky's death, when Australian student Kristi Kafcaloudis, 24, lost her balance and fell to her death. Ironically, Kafcaloudis was not taking a photograph or a selfie when she slipped and fell, but was waiting near the base of the tongue for two friends who had gone further out. [2.33]

Let's be clear: headline writers love drama, and the combination of "selfie" and "death" are simply irresistible to most. Clearly, people who are expecting a child or who would like to be expecting one someday should exercise some common sense about the types of photos they try to take and where they try to take them.

On a day-by-day basis, however, it is the distraction that devices can cause as we go about our daily lives that pose the greatest physical threat to our reproductive capabilities. Every time we move around in the world, whether on foot or by car, we should be focusing on where we are going and how we are getting there. The evidence is overwhelming that digital devices profoundly interfere with our ability to do so safely. If becoming a parent or continuing to be one is important to you, then put your device down and keep your head up.

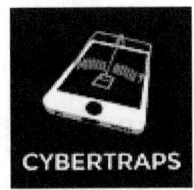

Chapter Three

Love Me Tinder, Love Me True:
The Impact of Geo-Social Dating Apps

Thirty years ago, in the film "Top Gun," a cocky Navy fighter pilot with the codename "Maverick" (played, it goes without saying, by Tom Cruise) strode into a San Diego bar called Kansas City Barbecue and said to his wingman "Goose" (Anthony Edwards): "This is what I call a target-rich environment." [3.1] It is not difficult to imagine the sheer glee with which Maverick would embrace the dating possibilities in today's mobile world. [3.2]

Computers have been playing an increasingly active role in human matchmaking since at least December 1964, when a group of Harvard College students came up with the idea of using one of the school's powerful "electronic brains" to process dating questionnaires and for a $3 fee, find a perfect romantic match for love-lorn, socially-awkward, blind-date-averse classmates. [3.3] Over the past half-century, computer-aided dating has proven incredibly popular: It has become a billion-dollar-plus industry, and one recent study concluded that more than a third of U.S. marriages now begin through some type of online dating. The study also suggested that married couples who meet online are more satisfied with their marriages than those who met "through family, work, bars/clubs or blind dates." [3.4]

The Rise of Geo-Social Dating Apps

As is the case with virtually every technological innovation, the potential benefits of online dating and computerized matchmaking are tempered by some serious and quickly-growing social and public health concerns. Over the last decade, a powerful witch's brew of mobile technology, the Global Positioning System (GPS), and social media has brought an entirely new and slightly frightening level of impersonal efficiency to the phenomenon. Web sites that offer a catalog of possible mates who can be courted through email, phone calls, and awkward first dates are now almost quaint; the driving force behind new relationships today are a range of apps, known collectively as geo-social dating apps, that make it possible to find a potentially compatible long-term companion or equally horny sexual partner within a few hundred or a few dozen feet of where you are standing right now.

The granddaddy in this category is **Grindr**, which was launched in the spring of 2009. In an interview with Grindr founder Joel Simkhai, the British newspaper *The Independent* offered a somewhat snarky description of the app:

> Grindr shows you, using GPS technology down to the nearest few feet, the men in your vicinity looking to meet other men. Probably not to exchange recipes. Thus, in 2009, human civilization evolved (or regressed, according to where you lie on the prude to rude spectrum) to a point where one could immediately find the nearest gay, bi or greedy man looking for sex. [3.5]

Grindr attempted to extend its concept to heterosexual daters by developing and releasing **Blendr** in 2011. A year later, however, a new app stole Blendr's thundr. Known as **Tinder**, the app introduced a new concept into the world of dating: the "swipe."

The simple but powerful user interface innovation has proven so compelling that it not only has been implemented in a wide range of other apps, but has also become a type of social shorthand for approval and disapproval. A Tinder user can use the app to browse the profiles and uploaded photos of other Tinder users, which are listed for each user based on an algorithm that takes into account geo-location, mutual Facebook friends, and shared interests. A swipe across the screen to the **right** signifies that the user is interested in a particular profile; a swipe to the **left** signifies disinterest. [3.6] The creator of a right-swiped profile is not notified of the other user's interest, however, unless he or she also right-swipes on the same user's profile. Once two users have liked each other's profiles, they can exchange messages, view common connections and interests, browse each other's Instagram feeds, and of course, hook up.

One of Tinder's co-founders, Sean Rad, explained the idea behind the dating app to *Inc.* in May 2013:

> The idea for Tinder came along when I started thinking about the fact that there are a lot of great platforms that help us communicate with people we already know, but there isn't a way for me to meet new people. In the real world, you're either a hunter or you're being hunted. If you're a hunter, there's

constant rejection. And if you're hunted, you're constantly being bombarded. And the current solutions actually make these problems worse. With other dating apps, I can reach out to more people if I'm a hunter, and I can be hunted more easily. I never used those apps, none of my friends ever used those apps, and I couldn't understand why until that aha! moment happened. None of these apps were solving the fundamental problem. [3.7]

Notwithstanding the decidedly unromantic view of relationships that apparently inspired its development, Tinder has proven to be wildly successful. Within six months of its release, the technology media company TechCrunch named it the "Best New Startup of 2013." [3.8] Just two years later, Tinder was believed to have over 50 million users, who collectively swipe right or left **3.4 billion** times each day. Twenty-six million of those daily swipes result in matches between users, adding to the more than 10 billion matches that Tinder has made in the four years since its launch. [3.9]

The startling popularity of geo-social dating/hook-up apps — particularly among millennials, who make up nearly 80% of Tinder's user base [3.10] — is raising a number of significant social and public health issues.

A Dating Apocalypse?

The most prevalent concern was dramatically highlighted by *Vanity Fair* contributor Nancy Jo Sales in her September 2015 article entitled "Tinder and the Dawn of the 'Dating Apocalypse'." Through conversations with various clusters of young men and women, mostly in Manhattan, Sales attempted to illustrate just how thoroughly millennials have embraced the "predatory" ethos that Rad and his fellow Tinder creators infused into their app. [3.11].

> "Guys view everything as a competition," [Alex (a pseudonym)] elaborates with his deep, reassuring voice. "Who's slept with the best, hottest girls?" With these dating apps, he says, "you're always sort of prowling. You could talk to two or three girls at a bar and pick the best one, or you can swipe a couple hundred people a day — the sample size is so much larger. It's setting up two or three Tinder dates a week and, chances are, sleeping with all of them, so you could rack up 100 girls you've slept with in a year."

Based on her interviews and a sprinkling of data from various sources, Sales identified some depressing trends in contemporary romance: the endless pursuit of the new, a profound aversion to commitment, inherent misogyny, abrupt and increasingly coarse hookup requests, an overall decline in respect for women, and a discernible rise, as it were, in levels of erectile dysfunction among millennial men. For good measure, Sales even threw in an allusion to The Sixth Extinction, a 2014 book by Elizabeth Kolbert that posits that we are living in a "human-propelled" extinction-level event.

Sales concluded her dystopian account of contemporary dating by posing a series of plaintive questions:

> So where is this all going to go? What happens after you've come of age in the age of Tinder? Will people ever be satisfied with a sexual or even emotional commitment to one person? And does that matter? Can men and women ever find true intimacy in a world where communication is mediated by screens; or trust, when they know their partner has an array of other, easily accessible options?

The push-back against Sales's grim sociological conclusions was swift. As numerous commentators pointed out, geo-social dating apps like Grindr and Tinder did not create the so-called "hook-up culture." Casual and spontaneous sexual pairings have been a by-product of alcohol-lubricated social gatherings for centuries — think harvest celebrations, Renaissance fairs, taverns and bars, frats and sororities, Madison Avenue cocktail parties, Tailhook conventions, politician/lobbyist junkets, academic conferences, and so on.

Over at *Slate*, Amanda Marcotte criticized Sales for "unskeptically" incorporating the "male braggadocio" of her interviewees into her article and suggesting that "phones are making men act like pigs."

"But last time I was single," Marcotte said, "there was no such thing as a smartphone, much less a dating app, and you could still find at least a few men who thought women were good for nothing but sex. ... Gross dudes were not invented by apps." [3.12]

Similarly, *New York Magazine* writer Jesse Singal sliced and diced Sales's methodology at length. While conceding that "wandering around and talking to people is important," Singal pointed out that there is a significant risk of "confirmation bias" — *i.e.*, that the majority of the people willing to talk about their dating habits on Tinder are those who are using the apps in ways that supported Sales's premise that a "dating apocalypse" is underway. [3.13]

Singal took particular issue with Sales's dismissive treatment of a recent study published in May 2015 in the *Archives of Sexual Behavior* by Professors Jean Twenge, Ryne Sherman, and Brooke E. Wells. Among other things, the authors concluded that while millennials are more accepting of the idea of premarital sex and more willing to report having casual sexual encounters themselves, they actually are less promiscuous, in terms of actual number of sexual partners, than baby boomers. After allowing for various generational factors, the researchers estimated that a baby boomer born in the 1950's has had an average of 11.68 sexual partners; for similarly-aged millennials born in the 1980's, the figure is 8.26. [3.14]

While Sales's dire view of 21st century romance may have lacked rigorous empirical support, there is no question that her provocatively-titled article struck a nerve. Many people, like BBC presenter and historian Dr. Lucy Wolsey, bemoan the ease with which "bored singletons" can browse for meaningless one-night stands. [3.15]

"As we see in period dramas," Dr. Wolsey said, "it's when there are terrible obstacles between couples that romance thrives best." [3.16]

Some Legitimate Concerns

While it may be tempting to speculate, as Dr. Wolsey does, on the impact of geo-social dating apps on such classic works of fiction as *Pride and Prejudice*, much more research needs to be done to determine the actual sociological impact of these apps and dating Web sites on romance, marriage, and parenthood. There are a number of issues that particularly bear further examination.

Why Aren't Millennials Getting Married?

The declining rate of marriage among millennials is an indisputable trend. The *New York Times* recently reported that as of 2012, the number of married households had dropped to 50.5%, "a historic low." [3.17] Among Americans ages 25 and older, the Pew Research Center found, a record 23% have never married, and as many as a quarter of all millennials may never marry at all. Of course, as the Center noted, the fact that someone is not married does not mean that they are single; almost 25% of millennials in the 25-34 age bracket were cohabiting with a partner. [3.18] But as economists and anxious grandparents like to point out, there are costs to delaying or avoiding marriage. The hallowed institution provides better tax treatment, clearer and more firmly established parental and visitation rights, greater economic security, and a more stable environment in which to raise children. [3.19] It is also generally easier to conceive and bear children in one's twenties and thirties, as opposed to mid- to late forties.

Sales, to be fair, is hardly the only person who believes that the endless choices offered by dating apps is partly to blame for the apparent disinterest of millennials in marriage. In an article cheerfully entitled "Tinder Is Tearing Society Apart," conservative *New York Post* columnist Naomi Schaefer Riley used Sales's article to go on a lengthy rant about the destructive impact of geo-social dating apps and the resulting hook-up culture.

"[I]f a critical mass of women are willing to be used by hook-up culture," Riley argued, "because that's what all the kids are doing these days, it affects everyone's prospects. Men too are allowed to live in a perpetual adolescence and never find out what it means to put effort into a relationship." [3.20]

Author and sociologist Eric Klinenberg agreed, telling the *Washington Post*: "The dating culture has changed. There's been a fundamental shift in the way people meet and find romance. Or even the way people in relationships communicate, due to technology." Klinenberg rejected the idea that dating apps will keep millennials single forever, but conceded that they can help millennials stay "very busy" when they're single. [3.21]

And predictably, in the weeks following the publication of Sales's article, *Cosmopolitan* went in search of married couples who first met on Tinder. It profiled four couples in a February 2016 article entitled "I Met My Husband on Tinder." The intro to the article nicely captures the challenges of the contemporary dating scene:

> Tinder can be such a horrific landscape of crotch shots and misspelled "compliments" about the way your breasts look in your profile pic that it's hard to believe anyone has actually met a life partner on there. But it happens. Cosmopolitan.com spoke with four women who found everything they were looking for in the place the last place they expected to find it: Tinder.

The Silence of the Nurseries

So perhaps the apocalypse is not fully upon us. But, wait, there's more: Another significant and disconcerting trend is that millennials in the

United States and in several other industrialized nations appear to be having significantly fewer children than previous generations. The National Center for Health Statistics reported that the overall U.S. fertility rate also hit an all-time low in 2013: just over 60 births per 1,000 women, or a total of 3.93 million births. The pregnancy rates for the majority of millennial women (those aged 15-29 in 2013) all showed declines over the last eight years. [3.22]

Undoubtedly, economic considerations play a far more significant role in a woman's or couple's decision to have a child than the rise of geo-social dating apps; the last decade has not been especially propitious for those thinking of starting or expanding a family. But in an era in which "courtship" is increasingly defined by emoji-filled booty texts, it is fair to wonder if the mobile dating revolution might be having a prophylactic effect as well.

It may also be true that thanks to social media, we are simply too busy and too self-absorbed to have children. By "we," of course, I mean people 25+ years younger than I am. A widely-touted recent study in England and Wales found that the rate of pregnancies among teenage girls has dropped 45 percent since 2007, when social media really began to take off, and are at their lowest levels in 50 years. [3.23] A lot of different possible explanations are being explored, including the most obvious: As teens spend more time socializing online, they spend less time in close physical proximity to each other, which reduces the potential for hanky-panky.

More Symptom than Cause?

It will take some time to determine whether social media and/or geo-social dating apps are in fact contributing to declining rates of marriage or childbearing. As we'll see in the next chapter, these are not the types of causal relationships that dating apps and social media sites find all that gratifying.

Frankly, I think that Sales and her like-minded colleagues have it backwards: Geo-social dating apps are not the cause of a dating apocalypse that is destroying marriage and parenthood. Instead, these apps are symptomatic of several much broader social trends that raise their own troubling issues. This one section may merit its own book someday, but here are a few brief thoughts about what drives the popularity of the mobile dating scene.

Too Many Choices

Vast amounts of server space are taken up with learned articles about the impact that the Internet has had on virtually every business or industry, from publishing to taxicabs to sex toys. All of them contain some variation on the word "disruptive." The chief reason that word is used so extensively is that over a twenty-plus year period, the World Wide Web has profoundly changed consumer expectations and behavior by vastly increasing both the amount information and the number of choices available to the public.

As comedian and actor Aziz Ansari pointed out, the overload of information and choices can make functioning in the modern world difficult. His parents, Ansari said, had an arranged marriage. His dad said he wanted to get married, his parents introduced him to three women, he spent 30 minutes talking to the third of them, they got married a week later, and have been together 35 years.

> Let's look at how I do things, maybe with a slightly less important decision, like the time I had to pick where to eat dinner in Seattle when I was on tour last year. First I texted four friends who travel and eat out a lot and whose judgment I trust. I checked the website Eater for its Heat Map, which includes new, tasty restaurants in the city. Then I checked Yelp. And GQ's online guide to Seattle. Finally I made my selection: Il Corvo, an Italian place that sounded amazing. Unfortunately, it was closed. (It only served lunch.) At that point I had run out of time because I had a show to do, so I ended up making a peanut-butter-and-banana sandwich on the bus. The stunning fact remained: it was quicker for my dad to find a wife than it is for me to decide where to eat dinner. [3.24]

The angst experienced by Ansari over a fairly simple question — where will I eat dinner? — is a variant of a broader social disorder affecting his generation. It's called FOMO ("fear of missing out") and it typically refers to seemingly overwhelming compulsion of smartphone users to check their devices constantly to what others have texted, posted, or photographed.

It can also refer to a corrosive sense of dissatisfaction with the choices one makes and the belief that with just a few more clicks or swipes, something better will appear. This is one of the impulses that underlies the use of mobile dating apps like Tinder and online sites like Ashley Madison. An analysis of Tinder users, for instance, found that 30 percent are married and another 12 percent are in a relationship; it will come as a shock to almost no one that the majority of those users are men. [3.25] And of course, the slogan of Ashley Madison plays directly into this: "Life Is Short. Have an Affair." As with so many other aspects of our lives, the seeming endless choices presented online leave us both overwhelmed and somehow unsatisfied at the same time.

Instant Gratification and the Death of Patience

Ironically, if we do actually get around to making a decision, our wishes can be gratified almost immediately. With the press of a button, we can download a powerful app that completely transforms how our phone operates, a two-hour movie we heard about a few months ago but never got around to watching, or a several-hundred page book. Earlier today, I realized that it had been some years since I read any of Sir Arthur Conan Doyle's great Sherlock Holmes stories. After a quick search on Amazon, I downloaded a complete copy of every single Holmes story for 99 cents, and it was delivered to my phone in seconds.

Physical objects don't take that much longer. An Uber cab will show up in 3-4 minutes, Seamless will deliver semi-hot take-out food in 30-40 minutes, and Amazon Prime Now promises to deliver your choice of tens of thousands of items with 1-2 hours if you live in a major urban area. How long will it be before drones and 3D-printing eliminate the tedium of even a 1-2 hour delay?

The stunning rapidity with which our consumer desires can be met is making us *significantly* less patient. According to a *New York Times* article from a few years ago, Google researchers discovered that "[p]eople will visit a Web site less often if it is slower than a close competitor by more than 250 milliseconds (a millisecond is a thousandth of a second)." [3.26] By comparison, it takes 400 milliseconds to blink once, and 417 milliseconds for a 99 mph fastball to reach home plate.

Is it any surprise, then, that the generations who have literally grown up with the Internet and mobile devices — millennials and Gen Z'ers — are drawn to mobile dating apps that offer seemingly endless sexual options and "relationships" that take less time than a pizza delivery? If a "dating apocalypse" is actually occurring, Tinder and its ilk are not the cause of it. They may well, however, be the proverbial canary in the coal mine for a society that doesn't know what it wants and is unwilling to wait for it anyway.

There doesn't seem to any serious concern that people will stop having children. After all, the procreative impulse is very powerful. Nor does it seem likely that the institution of marriage will entirely fade away. But it is also indisputably true that the central requirements of parenthood and marriage — patience, durability, fortitude, humor, resilience, sanguinity, and patience — are not qualities commonly reinforced by our digital distractions. If anything, most of the significant technology trends are destructive to the strength and stability of long-term relationships. Unfortunately, there are no easy answers for the next generation of expecting moms and dads; the single best solution is to be aware of the relationship challenges posed by technology and to discuss them as openly and honestly as possible.

To help spark that conversation, we need is a millennial Nora Ephron to write *You've Got Text* to help us sort it all out. In the meantime, these apt observations on pre-Tinder courtship by Jane Austen in <u>Pride and Prejudice</u> may offer some guidance to today's texters and Snapchatters (the emphasis is mine):

> "You are mistaken, Mr. Darcy, if you suppose that the *mode* of your declaration affected me in any other way, than as it spared the concern which I might have felt in refusing you, had you behaved in a more gentleman-like manner."

> "How little of permanent happiness could belong to a couple who were only brought together because their *passions* were stronger than their virtue."

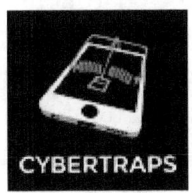

CYBERTRAPS

Chapter Four

"A Digital Bathhouse for Millennials"

Even if you don't view today's hook-up culture as the full-blown "dating apocalypse" described by *Vanity Fair*, there is one geo-social cybertrap that should be of concern to ***anyone*** who uses a mobile dating app, and particularly to those who either are pregnant or are contemplating getting pregnant at some point in the future.

The Rise in Geo-Socially Transmitted Infections

Over the last several years, public health organizations around the world have been raising alarms about an increase in sexually-transmitted infections among users of geo-social dating apps. One of the earliest reports appeared in 2014, following an investigation by a team of researchers among gay app users in Los Angeles County. The authors concluded: "sexual health clinic MSM ("men having sex with men") attendees who are meeting on GSN [geo-social networking] apps are at greater risk for gonorrhea and chlamydia than MSM attendees who meet in-person or on the Internet. Future interventions should explore the use of these novel technologies for testing promotion, prevention and education." [4.1]

Similarly, the Rhode Island Department of Health (RIDOH) issued a report in May 2015 that warned state residents of startling increases in the rates of infection by the human immunodeficiency virus (HIV) and a number of other sexually transmitted infections. Between 2013 and 2014, the number of infectious syphilis cases in the state rose by 79%, while the number of gonorrhea and HIV cases each increased by a third. RIDOH noted that the increased levels of infection were consistent with national statistics. [4.2]

> The increase [in rates of STDs] has been attributed to better testing by providers and to high-risk behaviors that have become more common in recent years. High-risk behaviors include using social media to arrange casual and often anonymous sexual encounters, having sex without a condom, having multiple sex partners, and having sex while under the

influence of drugs or alcohol.

Earlier this spring, the Canadian province of Alberta also argued that there is a link between social media and STIs, with officials saying that some infection rates were as high as they were in the 1980s at the height of the AIDS crisis. Cases of gonorrhea, for instance, rose 80 percent between 2014 and 2015, while the number of syphilis cases more than doubled. The two demographic categories that show the sharpest spikes were men who have sex with other men and women ages 15-24.

Another problem, Canadian officials said, is that some dating sites and apps effectively promote anonymous sex, since users don's have to enter accurate identifying information to set up an account. "When people don't know their sexual partner's identity," said Dr. Karen Grimsrud, the Alberta Chief Medical Officer of Health, "that makes it difficult for public health to do the tracing for them and their contact, as far as setting up testing and treatment." [4.3]

In England, Dr. Peter Greenhouse, a sexual health consultant for the National Health Service, warned of the potential for an "explosion of HIV in the heterosexual population." In 2014, the United Kingdom recorded a 33% increase in syphilis cases and a 19% increase in gonorrhea cases. [4.4] One publication promptly derided Dr. Greenhouse's opinion as a "Luddite view," and argued that the problem instead lies in better testing and a failure of the Government and families to provide adequate sex education to young people. Dr. Greenhouse later clarified his comments: "The tech is not to blame, the tech merely facilitates something that people wanted to do anyway. But the fact that the tech exists means that it's easier." [4.5]

Marie Cosnard, spokesperson for **Happn**, one of the United Kingdom's most popular dating apps, strenuously pushed back against Dr. Greenhouse's warning:

> Dating apps are following wider social trends and changing behaviors that have been unfolding for decades. There's a liberalization of attitudes towards the number of partners, the status of relationships, towards marriage, divorce, etc. So the rise of any STI is not really connected to dating apps themselves. The problem is much wider. People need to be more educated in terms of sexual health and to take their responsibilities, no matter how and where they've met their partner. [4.6]

It is certainly true that better sex education in the home and at all levels of education would help us make significant strides in reducing some of the less pleasant consequences of sex, from unwanted pregnancies to STIs. At the same time, it would be irresponsible for health organizations not to raise concerns about a potentially deadly link between geo-social dating apps and sexually transmitted infections. Whether coincidence or causation, graphs of the sharp increases in some sexually transmitted infections have a very similar shape to graphs showing the rise in the number of people using geo-social dating apps.

The debate over a possible connection got a little heated in late 2015, when the AIDS Healthcare Foundation (AHF) launched a billboard campaign in Los Angeles to warn of the dangers. The press release issued by AHF to announce its campaign referenced, among other things, Sales's article in *Vanity Fair*, as well as the health reports discussed above. [4.7] The campaign, which AHF said was featured on 20 area billboards and 100 bus benches, showed the silhouettes of two couples facing each other; the two individuals on the left were tagged with "tinder" and "chlamydia," while the two on the right were marked with "Grindr" and "gonorrhea." At the far right of the image was a URL, "freeSTDcheck.org." [4.8]

AHF President Michael Weinstein offered a powerful rationale for the organization's information campaign:

> Mobile dating apps are rapidly altering the sexual landscape by making casual sex as easily available as ordering a pizza. In many ways, location-based mobile dating apps are becoming a digital bathhouse for Millennials wherein the next sexual encounter can literally just be a few feet away — as well as the next STD. While these sexual encounters are often intentionally brief or even anonymous, sexually transmitted diseases can have lasting effects on an individual's personal health and can certainly create epidemics in communities at large. We want to send a strong message that sexually active adults — especially young people — should think twice about who they're hooking up with. [4.9]

Not surprisingly, Tinder and Grindr objected strenuously to the suggestion that there is a any connection between the use of their apps and the contraction of a sexually transmitted infection. [4.10] In a letter to Weinstein, Tinder attorney Jonathan Reichman described the billboards as "unprovoked and wholly unsubstantiated accusations" that were made by

AHF in an attempt to direct people to the organization's free STD test. He asserted that the advertising campaign, among other things, amounted to "false advertising, unfair competition and dilution by tarnishment" of Tinder's brand identity. [4.11] Weinstein dismissed Tinder's response as "tone deaf." [4.12]

Despite the stern tone of Reichman' letter, in early January 2016 Tinder added a new feature to its app: a "Health Safety" section that among other things, gives users the ability to search Healthvana.com to find the location of the nearest facility offering free STD tests. [4.13] The app change was announced in a press release issued jointly by Tinder, Healthvana, and AHF, along with the news that AHF would discontinue its billboard campaign.

"[I]t is such welcome news that Tinder will add a Health Safety section with a link to Healthvana, making it easier for people to find testing locations through an easily accessible, modern platform," said Whitney Engeran Cordova, the Senior Director for the AHF Public Health Division. "And we hope to see other dating sites do the same." [4.14]

In an email interview, Healthvana CEO Ramin Bastani praised Tinder for its decision: "Healthvana empowers people with their health information at their fingertips so they can make more informed decisions. The ability to have a transparent conversation about your health and test results before getting involved sexually is a good thing. The Tinder collaboration has potentially led millions of online daters to learn about their sexual health and give them resources to seek free HIV and STD testing." [4.15]

It's worth pointing out that what smartphone apps and social media giveth in terms of infection, they can also taketh away. There is tremendous potential in what one medical correspondent described as "crowd-sourced epidemiology." A number of different health and data organizations have been exploring ways to predict outbreaks of illness based on social media and other online information. [4.16] Beginning in November 2008, for instance, Google published "Google Flu Trends," which examined "aggregated search queries" to detect outbreaks of influenza across the United States.

> We compared these aggregated queries against data provided by the U.S. Centers for Disease Control and Prevention (CDC), and we found that there's a very close relationship between the frequency of these search queries and the number of people who are experiencing flu-like symptoms each week. As a result, if

we tally each day's flu-related search queries, we can estimate how many people have a flu-like illness. [4.17]

Another approach is to give people the opportunity to voluntarily report whether they are feeling any flu-like symptoms. The leader among that type of app is **flu near you**. After you sign up for an account and log into the app, you are given the chance to report on whether you are experiencing one of ten different symptoms, ranging from headache to nausea/vomiting. The app then transmits the data to epidemiologists working for Harvard University, Boston Children's Hospital, and the Skoll Global Threats Fund, where it is analyzed and collated with reports from other users. A map in the app shows reports in your area and assesses the risk of flu.

The Impact of STIs on Conception and Pregnancy

It will be great if crowd-sourcing epidemiology leads to faster and more effective responses to disease outbreaks. But if, as the evidence strongly suggests, geo-social dating apps are actively contributing to a rise in the number of sexually transmitted infections, then this is an issue that any expecting mom or dad should take seriously. Again, I am using the word "expecting" in the broadest possible sense to include not only those who are expecting a child right now but also those who may want to do so in the future.

Let me make one thing perfectly clear: My expertise is legal and technical, not medical, so while I hope that the following information is useful, it is *not a substitute* for talking with a qualified medical professional. Given the amount of well-researched, well-organized information available online about all of these issues, it may be tempting to do your own medical evaluation and diagnosis; again, what you read online is also *not a substitute* for talking with a qualified medical professional.

The evidence is absolutely unequivocal, however, that sexually transmitted infections, particularly if left untreated, can damage both male and female fertility, cause complications during pregnancy, and affect the health of your unborn child. *If you have any questions about any of this, or any concerns about your health, it is imperative that you consult your health care provider as soon as possible.*

Fertility and Conception

The first and most immediate consequence of a geo-socially

transmitted infection is the threat to your fertility and your ability to conceive. These critical aspects of human reproduction are fairly basic concepts but a review might be helpful: *Fertility* is defined as "the ability to produce young" [4.18], while *Conception* is defined as "the process of becoming pregnant involving fertilization or implantation or both." [4.19] Depending on its severity, a sexually transmitted infection can interfere with either or both of these critical aspects of reproduction.

Under the best of circumstances, conception is a dicey proposition. On average, a couple having unprotected sex has a 15 to 25 percent chance of getting pregnant in any given month. Those odds can be raised or lowered by a wide range of different factors, including but not limited to the age of the individuals involved, the frequency of intercourse, the positions used, the foods eaten, and of course, the health of each individual's reproductive cells. [4.20]

Public health officials worry about increases in infection rates because STIs can damage both sperm and ova. There is some research, for instance, that suggests that certain STIs — most notably HIV and chlamydia — can decrease the amount of sperm an infected male produces; HIV and chlamydia may also reduce a male's percentage of motile sperm, cells capable of propelling themselves through the uterus to the fallopian tubes. The lower the percentage of good swimmers, the lower the likelihood of fertilization. [4.21] More typically, STIs like gonorrhea and chlamydia diminish the fertility of infected males by causing scarring in the ejaculatory ducts and/or urethra of the penis, which physically prevents or limits the release of sperm. [4.22]

As is so often the case when it comes to human reproduction, the potential impact of STIs falls more heavily on women than on men. A woman's fallopian tubes, the tiny 4-inch organs that carry an ovum from the ovary to the uterus, are particularly vulnerable to genital infections. If left untreated, for instance, the STIs chlamydia or gonorrhea can cause inflammation described generally as "pelvic inflammatory disease" (PID). This inflammation can result in direct damage to the ovaries and the scarring of the fallopian tubes, which in turn can prevent sperm from reaching an ovum or can block a fertilized ovum from traveling into the uterus. In extreme circumstances, blocked fallopian tubes can result in an ectopic pregnancy, a nonviable pregnancy that poses a serious and possibly fatal health risk to the mother. [4.23] Public health officials are not kidding around when they say that this is a significant public health issue: More than a million women each year are treated for PID, and as many as 100,000 wind up completely infertile. [4.24]

Another STI that poses risks for female fertility is the human papillovirus (HPV). Unlike chlamydia or gonorrhea, HPV does not lead to pelvic inflammatory disease or directly threaten the female reproductive system. Instead, the threat to fertility and conception lies in the fact that HPV can cause cervical cancer; the side effects from the chemotherapy or radiation used to treat the cancer or in extreme cases, a medically-required hysterectomy, can destroy a woman's ability to bear children. [4.25]

Pregnancy and Health of the Fetus

The risks and potential consequences of STIs, geo-socially transmitted or not, do not disappear the instant conception successfully occurs. As the Centers for Disease Control point out, pregnancy does not create a magical shield against STIs. If you are pregnant or are planning to get pregnant, both you and your partner should be tested for STIs as part of your routine pregnancy care. [4.26] Many STIs do not have obvious symptoms or can lie dormant for a long period of time before manifesting themselves; nonetheless, they can complicate your pregnancy and potentially harm the fetus or newborn. [4.27]

Among the possible pregnancy complications arising from STIs are miscarriage or stillbirth (syphilis), illnesses and birth defects in the newborn (chlamydia, gonorrhea, genital herpes), and infection of the newborn (genital herpes, Hepatitis B, HIV). [4.28] As the CDC points out, some STIs can be treated during pregnancy, but unfortunately, not all:

> [STIs], such as chlamydia, gonorrhea, syphilis, trichomoniasis and BV can all be treated and cured with antibiotics that are safe to take during pregnancy. [STIs] that are caused by viruses, like genital herpes, hepatitis B, or HIV cannot be cured. However, in some cases these infections can be treated with antiviral medications or other preventive measures to reduce the risk of passing the infection to your baby. [4.29]

It's Time to Talk

Better Safe than Sorry

Notwithstanding the protestations of Tinder, Grindr, and other geo-social dating apps, the evidence appears to be increasingly clear that indiscriminate use of mobile dating apps is medically risky, unless everyone is practicing safe sex. That does not mean that people have to stop using them, of course. Like Tinder, some dating apps are starting to warn users about the potential risks and offer both safe sex advice and access to testing services. Those are important and valuable improvements to these apps, and it shouldn't have take this long for the information to be offered.

Of course, it is important to remember that neither social media nor geo-social dating apps are directly responsible for STIs, nor are they directly responsible for any stupid decisions made by their users. Most of these diseases have been around for centuries, and we know now that bacterial and viral transmissions occur because of a failure to practice safe sex. Infection has nothing to do with how two people met but is entirely dependent on their health and how they interact with each other. If anyone needs a quick refresher course, Planned Parenthood offers <u>a detailed overview</u> of the risks and how best to avoid them. The TL;DR version? *Always* use protection, until both you and your partner are in an honestly monogamous relationship and each of you knows the other's health status. That does not necessarily mean STI-free, of course; there are a growing number of dating apps that specifically cater to individuals with various STIs.

Trust Your Health Care Provider

It's also important to be honest and forthcoming with your health care provider, particularly if you are discussing pregnancy. If you've been using dating apps to go on a sexual bendr, it may be an embarrassing conversation, but it's not a time for false modesty. After all, you're not simply discussing your own health but potentially that of a brand new person who is entitled to the healthiest possible start to his or her life.

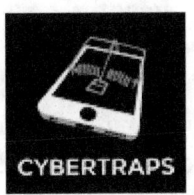

Chapter Five

Has Technology Ruined Sex?

The Centers for Disease Control and Prevention report that in the year 2014, there were 3,988,076 births in the United States. [5.1] That's a pretty impressive number. But spend some time researching trends in technology and sexuality, and you really do begin to wonder exactly where all of those babies came from. There is nothing headline writers love more than to declare in bold letters that "something" has "ruined sex." Among the leading culprits these days are: Netflix, "Game of Thrones," binging on box sets, Spotify(?), your dog, porn, sugar, Instagram, and of course, your smartphone.

It's a miracle we have any children at all.

The evidence is unequivocally clear that the seductive combination of technology and sex has a dark side; well, several, actually. Any one of the following tech challenges can pose problems for expecting moms and dads; taken together, they raise interesting sociological questions about the willingness or, in some cases, even the ability of millennials to choose parenthood over the endless pursuit of new Twitter and Instagram followers and rare Pokémon Go characters.

Distracted Intimacy

We've already seen the physical threats that distracted driving and distracted walking pose to our reproductive capabilities. A slower and more insidious threat, however, arises from the fact that technology is rapidly becoming a modern bundling board for device-addicted couples. We are bringing the entire world into our bedrooms and it's getting a bit crowded.

One of the ironies of the smartphone and table era is that these are devices that were designed to facilitate communication. And of course, they generally do. We use them every single day to talk to people, to text, to chat, to share status updates on Facebook, to post photos to Instagram or Snapchat, and so on. But the reality is that all too often, these same devices can reduce or even eliminate the interpersonal communication that is so critical to the establishment and maintenance of a successful sexual and parenting relationship.

Psychiatrists routinely express concern about this trend. When someone is staring at a screen, they warn, they are taking their focus away from anyone else who might be in the room, such as a partner or a child. The time spent interacting with online friends or playing games is time that is simply not available for nurturing in-person relationships. And if we're not developing and nurturing intimacy, how much less likely is it that we will feel the intimacy necessary to start or maintain a family?

This trend has gotten a lot of attention over the last few years from the mainstream press, as these headlines illustrate:

- "Your smartphone may be powering down your relationship," CNN, January 10, 2013;
- "Are you 'in love' with your SMARTPHONE? 75% of women admit devices are ruining their relationships," *Daily Mail*, December 8, 2014;
- "Yes, your smartphone is hurting your love life: study," *Fortune*, September 30, 2015;
- "How Your Smartphone is Ruining Your Relationship," *Time*, April 28, 2016.

The typical concerns identified by researchers in these articles are both predictable and understandable. They found that for people in a close relationship, the mere presence of the other person's cell phone lowered the perceived quality of the relationship, the feelings of intimacy and empathy, and the level of interpersonal trust. [5.2] A study at Baylor University said that "partner phubbing," — which they defined as "the practice of zoning out or snubbing one's partner in order to focus on a smartphone" — caused depression in over a third of the other people in the relationship, and near a quarter said that the behavior caused problems for the relationship itself. [5.3] A more recent study at the University of Arizona found that much of the dissatisfaction felt by the partners of phone-obsessives was simple jealousy.

"It's not use [of the device]," said Matthew Lapierre, assistant professor in the department of communication at the University of Arizona, one of the study's co-authors, "it's the [partner's] psychological relationship to that device." [5.4]

So, are you jealous of your partner's smartphone? Have digital devices caused problems in your relationship? Does your partner's obsession with his or her digital devices make it more or less enticing to plan a family together? Is it interfering with your sex life?

The answers to those questions obviously will vary from couple to couple, but recent surveys do not paint a very encouraging picture of sex in the digital age, either in terms of frequency or quality. It was bad enough in the 1980s and 1990s, when one partner or the other, or both, for that matter, might stay up until the wee hours of the morning playing games on computers or gaming devices in another room. Today, of course, all of those distractions fit into the palm of our hands, which doesn't leave them free for more procreative activities.

Five years ago, the navigation company Telenav asked over 500 Americans what they would be willing to give up for a week instead of their smartphone. Thirty-three percent said that they would choose their smartphone over sex; interestingly, seven out of ten of the chastity choosers were female. [5.5] When you first read something like that, it's a little shocking. But this might be the explanation: according to research by the University College London, the frequency with which people ages 16-44 had sex each month declined 20% over a two-year period, from just over 6 times per month to just under 5, or roughly once a week. [5.6] On the other hand, those same millennials are spending the equivalent of nearly one day per week using their phones. [5.7]

To make matters worse, when sex does occur, it's apparently not engaging enough to override our obsession with our smartphones. 62% of women and 48% of men told a British company that they have interrupted sex with a partner to check their phones. [5.8] More recent figures are slightly more encouraging, with just one person in ten admitting to checking his or her phone during sex. [5.9]

There are some couples who have turned smartphone distraction into a form of sex play. But for most couples, it might make sense to follow the recommendation of condom manufacturer Durex, which recently ran a "Turn Off Turn On" ad campaign. The company invited several couples to its research labs and offered to show them a feature on their phone that could dramatically improve their sex lives: The "Off" button.

Health and Safety Risks

The bedroom difficulties posed by smartphones are not limited to distraction and sexual disinterest. With so many of us using our phones and other tech devices in bed, there are a variety of health and safety issues that you also should consider.

Sleep Deprivation (And Not in a Good Way)

The first and most obvious is the fact that we are ruining our sleep by spending so much time staring at a bright light at the end of each day. As NBC reported last summer, 95% of Americans use an electronic device — "TV, a computer, a phone or a tablet" — within an hour of falling asleep. At the same time, 85% of Americans report that they have trouble sleeping. There's a connection. [5.10] According to the National Sleep Foundation:

> There is robust scientific data documenting the role of light in promoting wakefulness. … [C]areful studies have shown that even our small electronic devices emit sufficient light to miscue the brain and promote wakefulness. As adults we are subject to these influences and our children are particularly susceptible. [5.11]

Not surprisingly, a lack of sleep is terrible for your sex life. Among the negative effects are: Decreased libido, reduced vaginal lubrication, erectile dysfunction, stress, and depression. [5.12]

Electronics companies are increasingly aware of the sleep problem, which explains why Apple among others has implemented a "Night Shift" feature, which automatically shifts the light emitted by its phone from the blue end of the spectrum to a warmer rose color. [5.13] It doesn't address the distraction issue, but as a devoted iPhone book reader, I can attest that the change is much easier on the eyes, as is the white-on-black "night mode" offered by most electronic book readers these days.

That's Too Hot!

Sleep deprivation is the most widespread and ongoing health issue posed by smartphones, but it's not the only one. In fortunately rare instances, there's the possibility that your phone might get you hot in all the wrong ways. There have been reports recently of smartphone batteries overheating and causing fires. In February 2016, for instance, the New York Police Department tweeted several photos of charred pillows from various incidents in the U.S. and the United Kingdom. [5.14]

David Berardesca, the fire chief in Hamden, CT, told a local news outlet that the problem arose when the smartphone was tucked under the pillow all night. "These devices need areas to be ventilated," Berardesca said. "It is recommended that you leave these type of devices on a hard surface so the heat can dissipate. The batteries heat up, they could melt —

in some cases, explode — and cause a fire." [5.15]

Smartphones are not the only technology-related fire risk. Any sex toy that can be plugged in or contains a battery is a potential fire hazard. As with smartphones, these incidents are rare but the possibility is disconcerting nonetheless. A couple of years ago, for instance, Reddit user princess-heya posted an alarming message to the subreddit TwoXChromosomes:

> Hi ladies! I plugged in my Hitachi magic wand today, and it sparked/had actual tiny FLAMES right where the cord meets the body of the wand. It burned the cord right off. Thankfully neither I nor my lady bits were injured but I need recommendations for a new massager/vibrator. Preferably one that doesn't spark or catch on fire... [5.16]

Another user, writing on a different forum, reported that a battery malfunction caused her Rabbit vibrator to melt: "[I]t got so hot using energizer batteries," she said, "that the controls completely melted and seemed to find a speed that I had never been able to find before. Unable to shut the thing off with it stuck on this 'hyper speed.'" [5.17]

It's unclear whether "Sahara" appreciated the irony that her Rabbit was overexcited by Energizer batteries.

Radiation

If you are concerned about the potential effects of RF radiation on your body in general and your reproductive systems in particular (*see* Chapter One), then you probably want to keep cellphones and other radiation-emitting devices out of the bedroom or at least as far from your bed as possible. The most obvious issues arise if you are using your smartphone to augment your sex play. Fortunately, there are many sex-related apps that don't require access to the Web in order to function properly — for instance, long lists of sexual positions, sexual massage guides, erotic truth-or-dare, *etc.* — which means that you can put your phone in airplane mode and still fool around. Most apps, however, do require a connection to the Internet to function, which means that the phone is constantly transmitting to your WiFi or to the nearest cell tower while you play. It will continue to do so after you fall asleep unless you remember to turn it completely off.

Until recently, radiation was not something you had to worry about when choosing a sex toy. That's not to say that there weren't a range of other health risks, including numbness and skin irritation from overuse, infections from inadequately cleaned toys, stubbornly lodged toys, breakage, and adverse chemical reactions. [5.18]

Even today, the vast majority of sex toys are self-contained and don't include any transmitting technology. However, concerns about electromagnetic radiation are becoming an issue for innovative sex toy manufacturers like Lioness, which has incorporated Bluetooth into its vibrator to transmit data to a user's smartphone. To its credit, the company has proactively addressed this topic in its Frequently Asked Questions:

> **Wait...will there be bluetooth in my vagina?**
> Nope. We know that there are a lot of people who don't like the idea of bluetooth being on while in use, so we made it so bluetooth automatically turns off when you use it. [5.19]

But not every company is taking the same careful approach. Most of the growing number of Bluetooth-equipped sexual aids for both men and women, chiefly vibrators and plugs, don't make any mention of the possible risks of putting a microwave-emitting device inside various orifices of the body. Instead, they focus primarily on the ability of users to control the buzzes and vibrations of the toy using a connected smartphone app. As the manufacturer of the "Jump Egg Sex Toy" promises on its Web site, "Suitable for travel, long trip, or those live separately with her lovers. No matter how far away you are, with an App, he can still satisfy your sexual pleasure." [5.20]

Privacy and Security Concerns

You'll need to decide for yourself whether the idea of using a "smart" toy or having your partner control your vibrator from a hotel room hundreds of miles away is so compelling that it outweighs some of the legitimate health questions that remain unanswered. One thing that is clear is that there is a lot of interest in bringing this capability, known as "teledildonics," to the sex toy market. Actually, according to Jonathan Plotzger, erstwhile Director of Marketing for the sex toy company Good Vibrations, remote-controlled products have been popular for nearly twenty years:

> We had WiFi in its infancy (as it were) - radio-controlled vibrating panties were big, it was like a remote control for your partner, so you could act from across the room or perhaps at a crowded party.

Other, more sophisticated remote toys were just starting to come on the market - ones that were controlled via the web, so partners who were in different cities (either due to travel or in a long-distance relationship) could control the actions of the remote toy.

In the late 1990s, the potential privacy concerns regarding the use of sex toys was much lower. Of far greater concern to customers, Plotzger said, was that Good Vibrations would keep their shopping and their predilections confidential:

The privacy concerns that were voiced to us had more to do with keeping their names protected (as well as financial info, naturally). I never heard anyone concerned about information collected by a programmable or remote toy. Possibly this is because the only info that could be collected by the toy would be 1. its mere existence; and 2. what pattern of stimulation was used (which is esoteric & not very useful, e.g. "she likes quick vibrations" or "he likes slow rhythms").

What mattered was that we were respectable professionals who could have above-board conversations about very private matters, and not judge them. Everyone is afraid of being judged. As the head of the buying office, I used to work in the call center sometimes to support the staff AND get a feel for customers' concerns (I often worked @ the stores, too); on my first day, I had 2 calls - back to back - from straight men who were afraid that their desire for anal play made them gay. Fear of gayness = probably the number one fear of straight men. I'm talking about GV customers here, not making generalizations about the general population ;-) [5.21]

The Internet, of course, changes everything. It's much less clear whether any company, even a socially conscious one like Good Vibrations, can assure consumers that the data collected by Internet-connected sex toys is protected. As we'll see repeatedly throughout this book, the data that you generate when you use the Internet, Web sites, social media, and smartphone apps is incredibly valuable. It's valuable to the company that collects it, to advertisers, to governments and government agencies, to researchers, divorce attorneys, and potentially to law enforcement. If you are using a sex toy or a sex-related smartphone app that generates or collects data about you or your bedroom activities, then you should take a minute to look up and read the company's privacy policy. If it doesn't exist, think about buying a different toy. If it is difficult or seemingly impossible to understand, then take a lawyer or law student friend out to lunch and have them walk you through it.

True, it might be a little embarrassing or amusing to explain why you want to better understand the privacy policy of your favorite sex app or toy, and you might not really care whether the data collected is shared with advertisers. But you might feel differently if you later decide to put even more confidential medical information into a conception or pregnancy app. It's a good habit to think proactively about protecting your data and whenever possible, to use devices and software sold by companies that have simple, clear, consumer-friendly privacy policies.

Privacy and data protection are the more significant, long-term concerns during pregnancy for expecting moms & dads, but the real head-line grabber in this section is the possibility that a hacker might seize control of your sex toy and cause it to do unexpected and potential harmful things. In early 2016, the software firm Trend Micro held a press conference at the CeBIT technology conference in Hanover, Germany, and demonstrated how an Internet-connected vibrator could be remotely activated by typing just a few lines of code. [5.22]

The possibility that some random basement-dweller in eastern Europe might try to hack your Internet-connected vibrator is obviously disturbing, but probably not all that life-altering. What is worth keeping in mind, however, is that in the months and years to come, Internet-connected sex toys will get steadily more sophisticated. They will collect not only more data, but increasingly personal data — information that goes well beyond whether you and your device are turned "on" or "off." For instance, some toys may record voice or video as part of their operation, material that could be highly embarrassing if it is seized by an unauthorized user or subpoenaed during a divorce trial.

Perhaps in response to the Trend Micro demonstration, an anonymous user of We-Vibe, a "smart" vibrator, filed a class action lawsuit in early September 2016 against the company for collecting and transmitting private data about her vibration preferences and device usage across the Internet to the company's servers. We-Vibe's terms of service disclosed that such collection and transmission took place, but the company said it would attempt to clarify its language and give people the opportunity to opt out. The company also said that it had no indication that any breach of customer data had occurred. [5.23]

Hardware and software manufacturers all need to do a better job of protecting the data that they handle, from the moment of collection to back-end storage. After all, a toy manufacturer's servers may be just as vulnerable as the Internet connection that your device uses. But consumers have an obligation to be at least as "smart" as their toys. We need to think long and hard about whether the benefits offered by these new devices are worth the potential privacy costs. More importantly, we need to continue to push for better privacy protections for every aspect of data collection, transmission, and storage.

The Cybertraps of Endless Porn

There is no disputing the fact that our society today is absolutely awash in pornography. While we have been carving and painting erotic and even sexually explicit images for thousands of years, what we think of as "pornography" — commercially-produced photography and video content of a sexual nature intended for sale to adults — has really only been around for about a hundred and fifty years. For much of that time, pornography wasn't so easy for adults to find, and even more difficult for children. Today, though, tens of millions of sexually explicit stories, photos, and videos are available at the click of a button to anyone, young or old, who has access to the Internet. The sad and disturbing reality is that a significant portion of those materials are extremely violent and profoundly misogynistic.

There is considerable debate about the effects that these materials are having on our society as a whole and on individual men and women. However, there are at least three different areas of concern that are specifically relevant to expecting moms and dads.

Porn-Induced Erectile Dysfunction

In her *Vanity Fair* article, Sales recounts a conversation that she had with a group of women in an off-campus house at the University of Delaware:

> They talk about how it's not uncommon for their hookups to lose their erections. It's a curious medical phenomenon, the increased erectile dysfunction in young males, which has been attributed to everything from chemicals in processed foods to the lack of intimacy in hookup sex.
>
> "If a guy can't get hard," Rebecca says, "and I have to say, that

happens a lot, they just act like it's the end of the world." [5.24]

While there were some legitimate quibbles with the anecdotal nature of Sales's article, there also is a serious, ongoing scientific debate about whether millennials are having a hard time getting it up. Some psychiatrists and sex therapists do report an increase in a condition they describe as "porn-induced erectile dysfunction" (PIED). In an interview with the Huffington Post Australia, relationship counselor and sex therapist Alinda Small reported that PIED was the most common complaint of patients in her practice:

> Basically, what happens is your dopamine levels get a kick when you have a 'novel' factor, and porn is the most novel factor of all. Once you get hooked, porn gets more and more extreme, and so people start upping the ante on it. It gets to such a point where the expectation of pleasure is so high, normal sex with a real life partner doesn't provide that same hit. It's not as novel, especially in a situation where, for instance, the guy is with a long-term girlfriend. In many cases they would actually prefer to be wanking alone because they get that hit. [5.25]

However, many of the claims that large numbers of millennials are suffering from PIED are themselves based on little more than anecdotal evidence. One 2013 peer-reviewed study did find that 26% of "new onset erectile dysfunction" cases involved men under the age of 40, but no specific conclusions were reached as to why that was occurring. [5.26]

Two years later, researchers at UCLA and Montreal's Concordia University published a paper in the journal *Sexual Medicine* that reached an opposite conclusion. Researchers found that "[m]ore hours viewing VSS (visual sexual stimuli) was related to stronger experienced sexual responses to VSS in the laboratory, was unrelated to erectile functioning with a partner, and was related to stronger desire for sex with a partner." [5.27] However, the researchers also pointed out that the subjects of the study self-reported their response to the visual stimuli they were shown and were not observed in any way by the researchers. [5.28] A more accurate study could be performed by using instrumentation, such as a penile plethysmograph, to measure arousal and the maintenance of an erection while viewing various types of VSS.

Notwithstanding the lack of hard scientific evidence about the existence of PIED, there is a growing movement to help men disconnect from pornography or at least to stop using it as a masturbatory aid.

Organizations like NoFap ("Get a New Grip on Life") and PornHelp offer a variety of different resources, ranging from self-help guides to 12-step programs modeled on Alcoholics Anonymous.

The Relationship Risks of Pornography

Even if viewing pornography and/or masturbating to it is not contributing to an epidemic of flaccidity among millennial men (or older men, for that matter), it can still cause problems for expecting moms and dads by having an adverse impact on both your physical and emotional relationship.

The physical issues arise because viewing pornography and masturbation tend to go hand-in-hand, particularly for men. Pornography is not a prerequisite to masturbation, of course; many different animal species indulge in self-gratification and presumably they are not looking at porn when they do so. [5.29] Masturbation is a perfectly normal and quite common human activity as well, [5.30] and is a part of many fulfilling sexual relationships among couples.

It can be problematic, however, if it is indulged in so frequently that it interferes with a couple's sexual relationship or with other aspects of a person's life. It can, at the very least, be a time-consuming hobby. [5.31] It is worth noting that there is research data to support the intuitive assumption that the increased availability of visual sexual stimuli (*i.e.*, online porn) has resulted in an increase in the practice of masturbation, although it is difficult to quantify precisely by how much. [5.32] If you or your partner feel that masturbation is interfering with your sexual relationship and reducing the likelihood of conception, then you should take a look at the resources referenced in the previous section or speak to your health care provider.

The emotional risk of porn consumption is similarly serious. There is the very real possibility that a non-viewing partner may see the use of porn as a form of romantic or sexual betrayal. That was one of the things that occurred to the software reviewer who tested out Naughty America's virtual reality porn offering: "How would my girlfriend react knowing what I'd been getting up to at work? At what point do you have to consider it cheating?"

In this day and age of endlessly available porn, that's an important conversation for a couple to have once their relationship starts to get serious. Is viewing pornography a betrayal, is it joint sex play, or is there a "don't ask, don't tell" policy in place? Are there limits to how often or how hardcore? Is there a point at which "virtual" crosses over into an unacceptable reality?

Given our societal reticence to discuss either sex in general or masturbation in particular, these are not easy conversations to have, but they can prevent a lot of misunderstanding down the road.

Porn and the Male Mind

The cybertraps of PIED and possible relationship damage are risks that arise for specific individuals and couples. On a much broader basis, there is the issue of what effect the widespread availability of pornography is having on men in general, and in particular, on their attitudes towards body image, sex, and women as a whole.

This is a long-running debate that gathered steam not long after *Playboy* first appeared in 1953, and it accelerated in the 1970s following the launch of the openly misogynistic *Hustler* in 1974. But at the height of their success, adult magazines were only selling a few million copies per month. By contrast, there are tens of millions of Web sites that provide access to virtually unlimited amounts of sexually explicit videos and images. Moreover, thanks to our inability to effectively determine the age of any given Internet user, it is all but impossible to prevent kids from getting access to these materials. A recent British report, for instance, found that over 25% of children aged 11 and 12 had viewed adult material online at least once, and 4% did so every day; by age 14, 94% of kids admitted seeing X-rated content. [5.33]

Some sociologists argue strenuously that unfettered access to porn is warping the male mind in several important respects. Most notably, Professor Gail Dines, who teaches sociology at Wheelock College, recently wrote in the *Washington Post* that porn is a "public health crisis," echoing language used by the Utah House of Representatives in a recent resolution.

> After 40 years of peer-reviewed research, scholars can say with confidence that porn is an industrial product that shapes how we think about gender, sexuality, relationships, intimacy, sexual violence and gender equality — for the worse. By taking a health-focused view of porn and recognizing its radiating impact not only on consumers but also on society at large, Utah's resolution simply reflects the latest research. [5.34]

Dines offers a laundry list of studies demonstrating porn's ill effects: rape or sexual assault ideation, sexual aggression, sexual harassment, support for violence against women, low self-esteem among female partners, sexual behavior at a younger age, distortion of attitudes regarding "normal" sexual activity, and warped views regarding female bodies.

On the opposite side of the debate are researchers like Professor Justin Lehmiller, a sex educator and researcher at Ball University. In an article last fall, he highlighted research published in the *Journal of Sex Research,* which studied the attitudes towards women of more than 25,000 Americans collected over a 35-year period. The study concluded that both male and female "porn watchers reported more positive attitudes toward women holding positions of power, toward women in the workplace and toward abortion." He also cited a study from the journal *Aggression and Violent Behavior* that concluded that "greater porn use was linked to *less* sexual violence, not more." [5.35]

Whether the credibility of Professor Lehmiller's article is undercut by the fact that it was originally published in *Playboy* is for readers to decide, but it shouldn't come as a surprise that there are deeply-held opinions regarding the possible effects of pornography on individuals and society as a whole. It is equally unsurprising that it can be very difficult to reach firm conclusions about the attitudes people hold, how they were formed, and how significant the role of pornography might be in their formation. And when you consider how constitutional law, politics, and ideology can influence the interpretation of whatever data is collected, it quickly becomes apparent why this is such a fraught topic.

At the same time, as someone who has researched and written on this subject for nearly twenty years, I think the following observations are incontrovertible: 1) Vastly larger amounts of sexually explicit material are available than at any time before in our history, and the amount is steadily increasing; 2) over that same time frame, adult content has gotten steadily more violent, more misogynistic, and utterly decontextualized from any sense of relationship; and 3) any child with access to a device connected to the Internet has access to the same material available to any adult, which means that children now have unprecedented access to sexually explicit content. It is worthwhile to design and implement studies to try to assess the impact of these developments but at an intuitive level, I think it completely justifiable to be worried about the societal impact of these trends.

What can or should expecting moms and dads do about this? At one level, not much; no individual nor pair of individuals is going to solve the broad social challenges poised by the online adult industry. But what future parents can do is think long and hard, well before a child is born, about how best to develop the critical thinking habits and open communication skills necessary to parent your child(ren) responsibly in a complicated world.

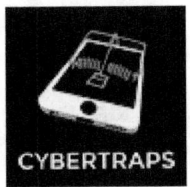

Chapter Six
Conception and Personal Privacy

More than 2,500 years ago, during his trial for impiety and corrupting the young, the Greek philosopher Socrates famously proclaimed that "the unexamined life is not worth living for human beings." [6.1] This was widely viewed as a defiant statement to the court that he had no intention of ceasing his self-described role as a gadfly in Athenian society. His clear lack of repentance contributed to the ensuing guilty verdict and a sentence of death by hemlock cocktail.

It's interesting to speculate on whether Socrates would think that the *over*examined life is worth living. In the two-plus decades since the popularization of the World Wide Web in 1993-95, the capacity of corporations and governments to collect and analyze data about every aspect of our lives — activities, interests, politics, hobbies, health, *etc.* — has absolutely exploded. Much of the damage to our privacy, of course, is selfie-inflicted, since we use digital devices (particularly smartphones) and social media to share ever-larger amounts of data about ourselves, our families, and our friends. And ever more rapidly, the so-called Internet of Things (IoT) is making it possible to capture data from any physical object to which sensors can be affixed. Thanks to rapid advances in miniaturization, that includes pretty much everything we can manufacture.

The collection of these vast mountains of data would be meaningless without the capability to store it and analyze it. Tremendous advances in server space and processing power are turning "data mining" into a multi-billion dollar industry that will fundamentally reshape many of our social institutions — manufacturing, marketing, health care, urban planning, anti-terrorism, politics, online dating, you name it.

We are only just beginning to assess the myriad ways in which data mining will challenge our concept of personal privacy. In the meantime, we should keep in mind another classical statement that is even more relevant today than it was when it was first penned over 2,000 years ago: *Quis custodiet ipsos custodes* ("Who will watch the watchmen?"). [6.2] What mechanisms can we put in place to better monitor what data is collected, how it is gathered, who has access to it, and how it will be used?

These questions are relevant to all aspects of a pregnancy, quite literally from the first moments of conception through birth and well beyond. In some cases, the collection of information about conception and pregnancy is purely accidental; more frequently, the efforts to acquire data about the progress of your pregnancy are highly purposeful. If there is one unalloyed truth when it comes to pregnancy, it is that all of the data associated with it — demographics about you and your partner, your health, the stages of your pregnancy, and so on — are valuable to an array of different entities, including governments, medical organizations, research institutions, and especially retailers of every description. After all, as *Parenting* magazine pointed out last year, you are likely to spend upwards of $20,000 on baby-related products and services before the little nipper turns one, and 7 or 8 times as much by the time your child hits 18. There's gold in your pregnancy-related data.

The Accidental Pregnancy Test

One of the many great things about the Internet is that it has facilitated the formation of an endless number of communities of people with similar interests, hobbies, politics, and passions. If there is something that you enjoy doing, the odds are overwhelming that you can find an online forum, chat group, or Web site to share your experiences and ask for help if you need assistance.

That's precisely what Reddit user YoungPTone decided to do in early February 2016, when his wife's Fitbit started acting oddly. YoungPTone (whose real name is David Trinidad) logged into the Fitbit subreddit and posted the following message:

> My wifes fitbit is showing her heartbeat being consistently high over the last few days. 2 days ago, a somewhat normal day, she logged 10 hours in the fat burning zone, which i would think to be impossible based on her activity level. Also her calories burned do seem accurate. I would imagine if she was in the the fat burning zone she would burn a ton of calories, so its not lining up.
> Im not sure if something is wrong with the sensor. is there a way to reset or recalibrate the device? Id like to try that before I contact customer service about a possible replacement. [6.3]

Among the responses to Trinidad's question was one from a user named ThatWasUnpleasant: "Has she experienced anything really stressful in the last few days or is it a possibility she is pregnant?" Trinidad wrote back: "pregnancy is a strong possibility, didnt know that would jack up the heart rate. I might be a dad, YIKES. now i gotta watch my own heart rate lol."

As he told the BBC a couple of days later, Trinidad called his wife and told her that she should take a pregnancy test. [6.4] She did and the couple discovered that they were in fact expecting. Not surprisingly, he posted the news to the Fitbit newsgroup:

> EDIT: Thank you all for your overwhelming support! Its been awesome to read all the comments and well wishes, even the comments questioning whether I am in fact the father (gotta have a sense of humor on here, right?). I just wanted to say this is indeed real, I do not work for fitbit, this is not guerrilla marketing. This is real, the fear is real, the excitement is very real! I am a regular guy who was just looking for the communities help with his wife's technology issue (we've all been there, right?). Little did i know I got alot more than I bargained for! Now I'm a regular guy who is preparing to have his first child brought into the world, god willing, in Oct 2016.

The as-yet-unborn infant is already something of an Internet presence: Trinidad and his wife Ivonne are posting periodic updates on both Instagram (@babyfitbit) and Twitter (@BabyFitBit). Later on in the book, I'll discuss some of the issues that raises, but for the moment, our focus is on the unintended by-product of Fitbit monitoring.

There is no suggestion that Fitbit was aware that its devices might alert female users to the fact that they are pregnant. On the other hand, the company is clearly devoting a lot of effort and research to better interpreting what people are doing when they wear its devices. For instance, in the latest firmware update, Fitbit devices gained the ability to automatically recognize six different types of exercise: walk, run, outdoor bike, elliptical, generic sports, and aerobic workout. Given the fact that Fitbit devices are already designed to record data about your sleep — last night, for instance, I slept 8 hours and 2 minutes, but was awake or restless for 21 minutes — how long will it be before these devices are capable to detecting and automatically recording when we have sex? That's clearly the type of thing that might be helpful for couples trying to conceive, particularly when paired with accurate information about the ovular cycle of the woman trying to conceive.

Fitbit devices are not the only sources of unexpected data regarding pregnancy and fertility. Remarkably enough, your cell phone bill also may offer some insights into those times when you are most fertile. Six years ago, researchers at the University of Miami analyzed the billing records of 48 women of child-bearing age. They charted the frequency with which the women called their fathers and their mothers, and then compared that chart to each woman's menstrual cycle. Their findings were fascinating: on average, the women called their fathers half as often during periods of high fertility and had much shorter conversations, regardless of who called whom.

The lead researcher, Dr. Debra Lieberman, suggested that the findings reflected evolutionary forces that discourage women from communicating during periods of high fertility with men who would be undesirable genetic mates:

> In humans, women are only fertile for a short window of time within their menstrual cycle. Sexual decisions during this time are critical as they could lead to pregnancy and the long-term commitment of raising a child. For this reason, it makes sense that women would reduce their interactions with male genetic relatives, who are undesirable mates. [6.5]

This is precisely what makes the explosion of data-collecting devices and services so fascinating. There is an insistent aspect to technological innovation, data collection, and data mining, and we simply don't know yet where all of this will take us. Perhaps Donald Rumsfeld, the Yogi Berra of the Defense Department, said it best:

> The message is that there are no 'knowns.' There are things we know that we know. There are known unknowns. That is to say there are things that we now know we don't know. But there are also unknown unknowns. There are things we do not know we don't know.

Although it was said in a much different context, that's actually a pretty good summary of the challenges of predicting what data mining will tell us about human behavior in the years to come. It's also a pretty decent summation of parenting as well.

A Digital Heads-Up for Prospective Parents

The heart-rate measuring capabilities of Fitbit and other activity monitors may not only help couples discover that they are pregnant, but may actually help them conceive. In 2000, British researchers determined that a woman's resting heart rate (RHR) accelerates as she begins to ovulate. In July 2016, Dr. Vedrana Hogqvist-Tabor, the scientific director for a fertility app manufacturer called Clue, published the results of a year-long study designed to determine if fitness devices equipped with heart rate monitors could provide early warning of ovulation. She and her team concluded that they "could give people at least 24 hrs of a peak fertile window notice." This was the first time, she said, that the earlier heart rate discovery had been tested with a readily-available consumer product. [6.6]

For Clue, the breakthrough linkage between heart-rate and Fitbit is an opportunity to carve out a bigger slice of the burgeoning market for fertility awareness method (FAM) apps. There are a large number of these apps in the iTunes and Google Play stores, all attempting to monetize the desires of some couples to become pregnant and others to avoid doing so. If Clue and its competitors are able to perfect the use of consumer heart rate monitoring as an accurate predictor for ovulation, it will represent a significant step forward in the often inexact estimation of a woman's peak fertility each month.

Not surprisingly, this is a subject that has been of more than passing interest to couples for a long, long time. The least scientific version of FAM is known as the rhythm method, which as millions of unsuccessful practitioners (also known as parents) can attest, is highly ineffectual. The rhythm method has probably been practiced on an informal basis for centuries, but it grew in popularity shortly before World War II, when researchers first published scientific data about average female menstrual cycles. [6.7] In 1932, an engineer named Gilmore Tillbrook invented a cardboard calculator called the "Rhythmeter" to help women determine their fertile days during each menstrual cycle. The wildly complicated-looking device should make us all appreciate the smartphone a little bit more.

Over the last half-century, our understanding of the biological indicia of ovulation has gotten significantly more nuanced. In addition to resting heart rate, other signs of ovulation include a change in a woman's basal body temperature, a change in the appearance of cervical fluid, and/or a shift in the appearance or firmness of the cervix. One of the challenges, however, as the American Pregnancy Association points out, is that most of the symptoms relating to ovulation vary from woman to woman, sometimes dramatically, and some women experience no symptoms whatsoever. [6.8] Hence the aggressive search for a combination of digital device and data collection that will provide a much more reliable and consistent prediction of fertility for each individual user.

A brief survey of some of the leading fertility apps [6.9] helps illustrate just how many different approaches there are even today for assisting women in predicting their most fertile days:

- **Fertility Friend** -- start and end of period, basal body temperature, cervical fluid observations, personal notes regarding mood and diet, medications, etc.;

- **Glow** -- ovulation and period calculator that uses data to get "smarter" over time; daily health logs of over 40 different symptoms; integrate data from Apple Health and fitness devices; the ability to add data for male partner;

- **Kindara** -- basal body temperature, cervical fluid observations, menstruation data, etc.; syncs via Bluetooth with electronic thermometer called Wink;

- **Clue** -- "31 tracking categories, including period, cramps, emotions, weight, skin, hair, sleep, exercise, weight, cravings, etc."; algorithm promises to make Clue more accurate in predicting cycle over time; in the process of being linked to fitness devices for heart rate;

- **Conceivable** -- "addresses 3 key areas that are scientifically proven to affect your ability to get and stay pregnant: your menstrual cycle, your lifestyle, and your ability to manage stress"; focuses on complete fertility wellness;

- **Period Tracker** -- "track period, moods, health symptoms, weight, temperature, weather, notes, medication, and pregnancy";

- **Ovia** -- allows users to track period and cycle, moods and physical systems, intercourse, weight and nutrition, sleep, ovulation tests and pregnancy tests, cervical fluid, activity and exercise, medications, blood pressure, and basal body temperature; syncs with fitness devices; claims algorithm generates most accurate predictions of cycle;

- **OvaCue** -- pairs with $299 OvaCue Mobile Fertility Monitor to help pinpoint most fertile days; tracks all menstrual cycle data; official charting app of Toni Weschler's book *Taking Charge of Your Fertility*;

- **Daysy** -- a $330 oral thermometer that assists women in predicting ovulation by measuring daily temperature and matching it to menstrual symptoms; using the "Lady-Comp" algorithm, it promises to predict ovulation and fertile days with 99.3% accuracy;

- **Natural Cycles** -- a monthly subscription service that uses a woman's daily temperature to predict fertile days; developers claim that their "complex algorithm" is 99% accurate in predicting the days in which a woman is fertile.

This rundown of fertility apps should make two things clear: First, even with all of our advances in technology, there are still aspects of human reproduction that are more uncertain than not. It may be, as the researchers at Clue hope, that a combination of data collection and data mining will eventually lead to insights that make predicting fertility less like the weather and more like actual lunar cycles. And second, all of these apps require users to enter highly personal data into a smartphone app, where it is stored and uploaded to the cloud for analysis. Of the two, it is the privacy issue that poses the most significant potential cybertraps for expecting moms and dads.

The Privacy of Conception

Limited HIPAA Protections

The data collected by the various fertility apps listed above illustrate one of the conundrums of personal privacy: In order to get better information or improved service, particularly with respect to health issues, it is typically necessary to disclose what most of us consider to be intensely private information. That's one of the reasons, of course, that Congress passed the Health Insurance Portability and Accountability Act (HIPAA) twenty years ago; among other things, it established "appropriate safeguards to protect the privacy of personal health information, and sets limits and conditions on the uses and disclosures that may be made of such information without patient authorization." [6.10] If you go to your physician for fertility advice or a pregnancy test, the doctor and the hospital may not release that information to anyone — the government, your employer, retailers, even your partner — without your express consent.

Unfortunately, the majority of fertility apps — and the companies that produce them — are not bound by HIPAA regulations but instead by much less stringent consumer privacy laws. The chief enforcement agency for consumer privacy in the United States is the Federal Trade

Commission (FTC), which has the power to take legal action to ensure that companies honor their promises to protect consumer information. Typically, this means that if a company lies about what they will do with consumer information, or if it fails to implement adequate security for sensitive information, the FTC can charge the company with a violation of the statutory prohibition against unfair and deceptive trade practices. [6.11]

To be fair, some of the leading fertility apps make fairly strong claims about protecting user privacy. Fertility Friend, for instance, unequivocally states that "Fertility Friend does not consider your data for sale or trade in any way. Your data is not a currency at Fertility Friend."

But other companies make users wade through multi-thousand word privacy statements written by lawyers for lawyers. The Kindara Web site, for instance, contains a fairly typical privacy statement, a 3,500-word tome that reads in part:

> Kindara (or its vendors and suppliers) may observe your activities, preferences, and transactional data (such as your IP address and browser type) as well as content you have viewed during your use of the Service. We may use this data for any purpose unless we tell you otherwise in connection with a particular Service. While we may collect or log this information, we do not identify you or match this non-Personal Information with your other Personal Information.

Kindara goes on to warn its users that it will use anonymized data for research purposes and that such anonymous data may be shared with third-party researchers. But, the company hastens to add, "Personal Information we share with a third party will be anonymous and not associated with your name or any identifying information provided by Kindara."

A Tempting Revenue Stream

Moreover, the health and personal data revealed by users is incredibly valuable, both in the aggregate and individually. The pools of data that apps like Glow and Kindara are compiling are obviously useful in helping women better understand their personal menstrual cycles, but they also hold enormous economic potential for the providers of fertility and pregnancy products and services, ranging from *in vitro* fertilization to vitamins to maternity clothing. (This is a topic I cover in more detail in Chapter Nine.)

In addition, the users of fertility apps tend to be Very Active Users; as one fertility app investor put it, some of these apps have "Candy Crush" levels of user engagement. It shouldn't come as a surprise, then, that this category of apps has been one of the most popular categories for venture capital. [6.12]

Given the fact that many of these fertility apps are free, it should come as no surprise that the companies that provide them are struggling to figure out how to generate the revenue needed to keep operating. To quote one of Gary Trudeau's myriad insightful "Doonesbury" cartoons, "But the pension fund was just sitting there." In a highly-competitive medical app marketplace, fertility app operators are perpetually teased by the fact that marketers and retailers will pay serious coin for the data just sitting on their servers. And the cold reality is that there is very little effective regulatory oversight as to how fertility app companies handle the data they collect.

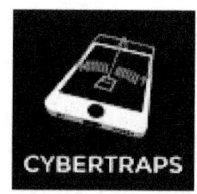

Section Two

The Cybertraps of Pregnancy

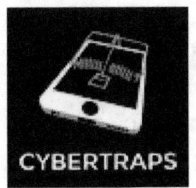

Chapter Seven

Social Media Risks at the Start of Pregnancy

A Digital Technology Plan

Towards the end of pregnancy, pediatricians and health organizations typically recommend that expecting mothers and couples sit down and write a birthing plan. The purpose of the birthing plan is to give you a chance to think through each step of the delivery process and write down your preferences for what you would ideally like to happen. For instance, you might want to think ahead about who should be in the birthing room, the labor positions you would like to use, what type of pain management should be provided, how warm or cool you'd like the room, the type of music you'd playing (if any), and so on. [7.1] You'll want to discuss each element of the birth plan with your physician or your midwife and make contingency plans in case things don't go as expected.

When a couple decides to start trying for a baby or discovers that one is on the way, one of the first things that they should do is to create a digital technology plan for the pregnancy. It can come as a shock to many young couples that they don't necessarily agree about every parenting issue that arises and that is almost certainly true as well for the use of digital technology during and after a pregnancy. In my experience, one person in a relationship tends to be much more technology-oriented or active on social media than the other and of course, each person is likely to have his or her own definition of what is or should be "private." If the mother of your child doesn't want photos of her in labor on Facebook, it's good to know that *before* her water breaks.

Couples can minimize unpleasant surprises and disagreements by taking a few minutes to talk through the issues that I discuss in the remainder of this book and make some preliminary decisions about what technology will be used during pregnancy, how much information will be shared on social media, who will share it, what services will be used, and who will have access to the data. Above all, you should think about the fact that you are no longer posting for just yourself or for the two of you, but also for a new human being who has implicit rights of self-determination that he or she will not be able to fully exercise for years to come. I'll return to this subject in more detail towards the end of the book, but it is definitely a topic that expecting parents should sort out between themselves early in a pregnancy.

The chapters and subheadings in the balance of the book will offer some guidelines for this discussion. To help facilitate the drafting of a digital technology pregnancy plan, I've also included a list of relevant topics and questions in Appendix A.

Urine My Facebook Feed?

One would think that something so intimate and precious as the conception of a child would be such a private experience that no one would think to share it on social media, particularly since the chief method for determining pregnancy at home involves peeing on a plastic stick. One, of course, would be sadly mistaken.

There is always a celebrity or two willing to over-share their personal lives on social media, even when it comes to pregnancy. In May 2016, for instance, Kim Kardashian was on an airplane and apparently had a bit of a panic attack over the possibility that she might be pregnant. She first sent out a Snapchat photo of three(!) different pregnancy tests, then shared a video in which she said ""I'm legit in the airplane bathroom, going to take a pregnancy test, because I'm having a little bit of a scare. So, no big deal." A few minutes later, she posted a photo of a ClearBlue pregnancy stick showing the words "Not Pregnant." [7.2]

While Kardashian may have been experiencing a moment of personal panic, executives at ClearBlue were undoubtedly doing cartwheels. The photo showing the negative result, with ClearBlue's label clearly displayed, attracted enormous media attention. Given the fact that Kardashian normally commands upwards of $1 million for brand endorsements, that's a pretty sweet publicity bump for the pregnancy test company. [7.3] Ironically, ClearBlue actually has been paying celebrities over the last several years to share photos of their pregnancy tests on social media; among those who agreed to ClearBlue sponsorship of their good news are Kendra Wilkinson, Melissa Rycroft, and most recently, Alex and Carlos PenaVega. [7.4]

The practice of sharing pregnancy stick test results on social media is not limited to celebrities, of course; a large number of non-celebrities do so as well. Social media is filled with pictures and videos of women sharing the results of their pregnancy test. A recent search, for instance, revealed that there are just under 400,000 "pregnancy test" videos on

YouTube. Many of the videos are posted to a channel on YouTube called "Womb Tube," which was created by blogger Rachel Eyre, editor of The Healthy Womb. As Slate writer Marisa Meltzer warns, "If the sight of urine makes you uncomfortable, WombTube is not for you." [7.5]

So here's your first digital technology pregnancy plan question: How do you and/or your partner feel about the idea of announcing your pregnancy by holding up a pee-soaked pregnancy test? Be prepared for the fact that if you decide to go that route, there will definitely be those who think it's tacky. Or as one blogger on the Web site Mommyish put it, "Posting A Positive Pregnancy Test On Social Media Is Gross, #SorryNotSorry." [7.6]

Beyond issues of good taste, there are other reasons why you might want to pause and think twice before broadcasting a photo or video of your pregnancy test. A particularly significant one is that you might not actually be pregnant. Consumer pregnancy tests are mainly based on detection of the human Chorionic Gonadoptropin (hCG) hormone in a woman's urine; blood can also be tested for hCG, but that is a less consumer-friendly option. The hormone is first detectable roughly 10-14 days after conception; it doubles every 36-48 hours thereafter for the first two months of pregnancy and then levels off. Home pregnancy tests require a woman to either dip a test strip in urine or pee directly on it; after a few minutes, depending on the specific brand, a results window will show either a line or a plus sign to indicate that hCG has been detected. [7.7]

Although pregnancy tests are accurate 90-95% of the time if done correctly, reading the results of a test strip is not an exact science. The darkness of lines in the results window is a rough indicator of the level of hCG in a woman's urine. So, in the very earliest days of a pregnancy, the line may be incredibly faint. In their eagerness to find out the results of their test at the earliest possible moment, many women use photo editing software like Photoshop to digitally manipulate a photograph of the pregnancy test. By tweaking contrast, brightness, and other elements of the photograph, it is sometimes is possible to "see" a positive result that is not visible to the naked eye. On various pregnancy and parenting forums, Photoshop-savvy women offer their editing services, and anxious would-be mothers upload photos for assistance and crowd-sourced test result interpretation. [7.8] For $1.99, you can even buy an app called "Early HPT+" that can assist in tweaking images of pregnancy test results on your smartphone.

Unfortunately, there are alternative explanation for a very faint line in a pregnancy test result: The stick could be defective or past its expiration date, or a woman might be experiencing what is called a *chemical pregnancy*, a phenomenon that characterizes as many as three-quarters of all miscarriages. The term refers to a miscarriage that occurs shortly after fertilization of an egg by a sperm cell; the only actual evidence of a pregnancy is the presence of trace amounts of hCG in blood and urine. [7.9]

Thanks to technology, the tweaking of pregnancy test result photos may soon be a thing of the past. Many of the photos and videos posted recently, including those shared by Kim Kardashian, show women using the ClearBlue Digital Pregnancy Test. The device has a countdown feature that shows you how much longer you have to wait and then reports the results by displaying the words "Pregnant" or "Not Pregnant." That certainly cuts down on the need for interpretation of faint lines. Presumably, digital pregnancy tests are programmed only to show the word "Pregnant" if your hCG is at a certain level, but there is no readily-available information regarding what actual concentration of hCG triggers a positive result.

Other Pregnancy Announcement Cybertraps

In these days of increasingly far-flung families, social media offers an incredibly efficient way to stay in touch with your family. Like so many others, I don't live within easy driving distance of my siblings and their kids, so Facebook and increasingly, Instagram, has been a great way to stay in touch and see the highlights of their day-to-day lives. And there's no arguing with the fact that social media is a highly effective way to share news with the various people who have drifted in and out of our lives over the decades.

But before you click on the blue-and-white "Post" button to share your happy news, there are a number of issues you should consider. Here's a sampling of things that you and your partner should discuss.

Are Pregnancy Announcements Just Tacky?

Social media is a sufficiently recent phenomenon that our cultural norms regarding its use are still evolving. Perhaps the first question is whether it is ever appropriate to use social media to announce a pregnancy. A few years ago, a woman named Buranda asked readers of a mother's forum called Mumsnet about "Announcing pregnancy on Facebook?" She admitted that she was conflicted: "I'm seriously in two minds about doing this. Part of me feels like it's really tacky, and quite a personal thing - and another part of me thinks it would be so much easier to let a huge amount of people know. What do you all think?" [7.10]

As you might expect, the answers from the other mums were all over the map. Many people suggested that it's too crass and impersonal, or even in unforgivably bad taste. Others valued the efficiency of letting a lot of people know at once and were thrilled to get the congratulations from their Facebook friends. Notwithstanding just how emphatic some people are about this issue, there really isn't a right answer. And given the fact that the vast majority of women of child-bearing age are millennials, who have grown up posting virtually every aspect of their lives online, it's likely that fewer and fewer people will object to the idea of a social media pregnancy announcement. If you need any reassurance on this point, do a search on Pinterest for "Facebook Pregnancy Announcement" — there are thousands of different ideas.

Too Soon?

But even if you and your partner agree that you'd like to spread the good word of your pregnancy on social media, there are still a couple of timing issues that should be considered. First, assuming that your pregnancy test is not already on social media, you and your partner will want to decide how quickly you want to tell anyone. Between 10% and 20% of all known pregnancies end in miscarriage and 80% of those involuntary terminations occur during the first 12 weeks of pregnancy. [7.11] That's why so many couples wait to share their good news until the first three months of a pregnancy have safely passed.

Second, you should think carefully about notifying the people close to you IRL (*in real life*) who should be told in person, by phone, or via video chat before your adorable social media announcement gets posted. Of course, given that everyone you tell in person is undoubtedly on social media themselves, you'll want to make it clear to everyone just how long the information should be embargoed. As one Mumsnet poster warned, that might include your partner:

> Bloody facebook, DH posted an update that we were expecting another baby before I had told everyone important, so a few people found out that way and I was mortified. Even though I told him to remove it literally an hour after posting (as soon as I found out) it was amazing how many people had already seen it. Avoid like the plague unless you are 100% certain that everyone

you want to tell in person has been told, and even then you have to ask them not to post anything on FB!! Arggghhhh! [7.12]

Whether "DH" is shorthand for "dear husband" or something much less flattering, it highlights the challenge of keeping *anything* secret these days. Obviously, there is a point at which a pregnancy announces itself, either to people in the same room with you or in photos, but you still are entitled to control what images of you are posted to social media. There's certainly no statutory requirement that you announce your pregnancy on social media, and there are some pretty compelling reasons to think twice about contributing to the absolutely staggering number of "baby bump" photos online. Type that phrase into Google, for instance, and you can choose from any one of 15.7 *million* different search results, many of which are galleries of photos of expecting mothers. More on that in a later chapter.

The Empathy Factor

One of the topics that is gaining increasing attention these days is the impact of technology on the development of empathy among young children. As I discussed earlier, scientists have documented a steady decline in self-reported feelings of empathy among college students over the last twenty years. I believe that anyone who uses social media or texting as a means of communication is at risk of decreased empathy when dealing with other people, which the rise of Internet trolls amply demonstrates. The simple truth of the matter is that when you cannot see someone's reactions in real time, your ability to understand the impact of your statements is greatly diminished.

Announcements of pregnancy offer a good example. Before the average person was handed the amazing broadcast capabilities of social media, the announcement of a significant life event like pregnancy was a much more carefully curated moment. Unless you were a bit of a misanthrope or worse, some sort of low-level sociopath, you would take the experiences and feelings of other people into account when you shared your news. So, for instance, if you knew that one of your friends had been trying to conceive for years or had recently had a miscarriage, you probably would tone down your excitement, find some way to filter your good news through an intermediary, or even just wait until there was no way to hide your pending arrival. But social media does not make it easy or even possible to be that discriminating about who among your friends sees your posts.

To be fair, people who are active on social media should realize that they run some risk that they will see posts that will upset them. Everyone has a responsibility to think about how they use social media and whether there are times when the costs outweigh the benefits. I'm certainly not suggesting that you can't or even that you shouldn't post the news of your pregnancy online. What I do think is important is to think about who might see the news and how it might affect them, and tailor your announcement accordingly.

How Do You Want Your Boss to Find Out?

There's one person you probably don't want learning about your pregnancy over social media: your employer. According to the Pew Research Center, just under two-thirds of women who gave birth between 2006 and 2008 (the latest available figures) were employed at least part-time during their pregnancy. [7.13] While most industrialized nations have adopted laws protecting pregnant women from employment discrimination, the reality is that the news of an impending birth will inevitably alter your workplace environment, from comments and questions by co-workers to concerns about time off for medical appointments to the types of assignments you are given. In 2015, the U.S. Supreme Court did make it slightly easier for pregnant women to challenge discriminatory workplace policies, but there are still a lot of unanswered questions about exactly what types of accommodations are required for expecting workers. [7.14] If you are employed when you learn that you are pregnant, then you should take time to do some research on your rights or consult with an attorney before things progress too far.

If your objective is to delay telling your employer as long as possible, then you really do need to think about whether it is advisable to post anything about your pregnancy on social media. Are any of your co-workers friends with you on Facebook or followers on Instagram or Snapchat? The odds are good that you are social media buddies with at least one co-worker, if not more. Even if your boss or supervisor is not among your immediate social media friends, he or she might be a friend of a friend, which would enable him or her to see what you posted. The information might also simply be passed on by one of your "friends," either electronically — since *anything* that is digitized can be copied and pasted — or the old-fashioned way, across a water cooler or in the company kitchen. In most instances, things will go more smoothly if you are the one delivering the news to your boss rather than some random chain of gossips.

Even after your colleagues and supervisors know that you are pregnant, it is important to think carefully about what you are sharing about your pregnancy on social media. While your siblings or your parents might be fascinated by the physical ups and downs of your pregnancy, your co-workers might be less enthused. That is particularly true, incidentally, if your social media profile identifies where you work, your position, or perhaps even the names of some of your clients.

There is a concept known as "siloing" that might be worth considering: it refers to the process of separating certain departments, agencies, or channels of information from one another. In the context of social media, siloing is used to differentiate where certain types of information is shared and with whom. For instance, you might use LinkedIn to share information about your work with professional contacts. Your Facebook account might be set up under an informal name (Jon instead of Jonathan, for instance) and not contain any information regarding your work. Your Instagram or Snapchat account might be a pseudonym or just a first name. You can then choose the appropriate channel for specific types of information: A photo of your fried dough lunch at the county fair could go on Snapchat, a summary of Thanksgiving might be appropriate for Facebook, and news of a promotion would be best suited for LinkedIn.

Make no mistake, however: While siloing information is a useful tool, it's not a perfect means of protecting your information. The only way to prevent information from spreading on social media is to keep the information *off* social media. Even the tightest and most carefully curated privacy settings will not protect you if one of your social media "friends" decides to copy something you've posted and share it either on their social media or in hard copy. As I described in *Cybertraps for Educators*, there are dozens of now-unemployed teachers who thought they were only sharing with friends, only to discover that their friends did not agree with what they said or what they shared.

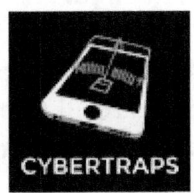

CYBERTRAPS

Chapter Eight
Technology and Health Risks to the Fetus

Once conception occurs and a fertilized egg implants itself in the uterus, a miraculous 9-month process begins. From the outset — and even beforehand, if possible — it is important to take reasonable steps to help protect the health and safety of your future child. Any competent pediatrician will provide you and your partner with a long list of dos and don'ts to promote a healthy and successful pregnancy, but here is a brief preview:

- Make healthy food choices;
- Take prenatal vitamins (particularly folic acid);
- Exercise regularly;
- Take sensible safety precautions (wear your seat belt and don't text!);
- Avoid hot tubs and saunas;
- Avoid unnecessary exposure to chemicals (the non-pregnant partner can clean for a few months);
- Get plenty of rest;
- Avoid alcohol, drugs, and tobacco;
- Monitor your weight gain;
- Limit caffeine intake; and
- Listen to your pediatrician or midwife.

What often gets overlooked, even by the most meticulous midwives or pediatricians, are the potential risks that the use of technology can pose to a pregnant woman and her unborn child. As with so many of the potential risks discussed in this book, there are varying levels of disagreement about the severity of the risk or whether it is a risk at all. At the very least, however, the following cybertraps are all important topics to discuss with your partner and with your health care provider(s).

The Internet Can Make You Crazy

One of the first things that people often do when they discover that they are pregnant, or are feeling ill in some way, is to log onto the Internet and start doing their own research. It's an understandable temptation: there are vast amounts of health-related information online and whatever your concerns, the odds are good that you can find a Web page or even an entire Web site stuffed with information. That's particularly true for pregnancy; there are an almost endless number of Web sites devoted to absolutely every aspect of pregnancy, from problems with conception to all-natural birthing techniques.

A study by doctors from the Mayo Clinic makes it clear, however, that attempts to self-diagnose are not likely to be successful. The researchers set out to answer a pretty straight-forward question: whether "symptom-related Web sites give sufficient information for users to seek urgent care when warranted." They concluded that the answer was largely "no."

> Of the 120 sites reviewed, 41 (33%) contained no critical symptom indicators. No site contained a complete set of critical symptom indicators. Overall, out of the 1,020 total critical symptoms searched for in the sites, we only found 329 (32%). When present, critical symptom indicators were found on the top half of the first page of the site in only 34%. Specific recommendations for further care were absent in 42% of the cases where critical symptom indicators were identified. [8.1]

To overcome the limitations of the self-directed Internet search, software developers have created "symptom checkers," which can be found both online and in the various app stores. These sites and apps use increasingly sophisticated lists of questions to help guide users to possible diagnoses and recommended care options. While symptom checkers generally offer better advice than self-diagnosis through Web searches, there is still significant room for improvement. Researchers who tested online symptom checkers reported that only one-third provided the correct diagnosis as the first choice, and less than two-thirds included it in the top twenty choices. Mobile apps did slightly better in identifying serious issues and recommending medical attention, but as one writer put it, that's because health-care apps are "biased towards advising patients to seek professional care even when self-care is appropriate." [8.2] That makes sense, of course, because no software company nor and of its lawyers want to run the liability risk of telling people they can self-treat when hospital care is required.

There are some who believe that if you throw enough processing power and data at a problem like health care, even better solutions will emerge. That's the general concept behind IBM Watson Health, which is attempting to harness the awesome power of the IBM Watson computer to provide faster and more accurate diagnoses. IBM prefers the term "cognitive computing" to "artificial intelligence," but to the end user, *i.e.,* patients, the distinction may not be all that meaningful. [8.3] What does seem fairly certain is that in the not-too-distant future, digital devices will be offering increasingly sophisticated and accurate answers to the question "What's wrong with me?"

In the meantime, the first cybertrap that arises during your pregnancy is the impulse to rely on the Internet for anything more than the most general medical information. Yes, it can be valuable to have an overall understanding of the issues that may arise during your pregnancy and it is certainly good to know what questions you should ask your health care provider, but avoid as much as possible plunging down the rabbit hole that is the Internet. And as we will shortly see, even if the possibility of inadequate or even incorrect information is not sufficiently disconcerting, the privacy risks should be.

You're Now Walking for Two

If you are pregnant or have recently discovered that you are pregnant, please be sure to read about the risks of digital distraction in Chapter Two. It turns out that driving while pregnant is already a high-risk activity, particularly during a woman's second trimester; a recent Canadian study concluded that women at that stage of their pregnancy are as likely to get in an accident as someone suffering from sleep apnea. [8.4]

There don't appear to be any studies that have researched the number of cellphone-distracted accidents, either driving or walking, that specifically involve pregnant women. The reality is that they are probably not needed: Cellphone use while driving and walking is dangerous to *everyone*, pregnant or not. It's just another precaution for women to keep in mind during the course of their parturiency.

Some Physical Phenomena to Consider

As I noted earlier, we are in the process of conducting a long-running experiment about the effects of mobile devices on our bodies. If you spend any time researching this on the Internet, you will quickly discover that opinions about this "experiment" run the full gamut of human opinion, from the tin-foil brigade to the Alfred E. Neuman acolytes ("What, Me

Worry?"). Where you fall on that spectrum is something you will need to decide for yourself, after discussing these issues thoroughly with your partner and your health care professional.

Regardless of what you ultimately decide, do your best to avoid endlessly researching these issues. That way madness lies.

Making Sound Decisions for Your Child

The impact of sound on your fetus or unborn child offers a good example of how difficult it is to balance competing issues when it comes to technology and pregnancy. More than twenty years ago, psychologist Frances Rauscher published a paper in which she reported that students who listed to ten minutes of a Mozart sonata in D-major performed significantly better on a spatial recognition test involving cuts to folded paper. Through some undetermined process of parental groupthink, that narrow finding launched a small cottage industry of books and music CDs for pregnant women, on the theory that exposing an unborn child to Mozart would ensure his or her later academic success. In 1998, Georgia governor Zell Miller launched a program, with funding from Sony, to distribute a classical music CD called "Build Your Baby's Brain — Through the Power of Music!," and Florida adopted a regulation requiring daycare centers to play classical symphonies on their sound systems. [8.5]

As well-intentioned as that all was, there is just one small problem: Researchers have had a hard enough time replicating the so-called "Mozart effect" among origami-challenged college students, let alone assessing the impact on the rapidly-developing brains of fetuses. There have been studies that suggest that playing classical music after the fourth month of pregnancy can in fact assist in the development of neural bridges within the brain and can help foster a sense of calm for the fetus. [8.6] But more recent investigations find no evidence that prenatal Mozart sessions have any long-lasting impact on intelligence. Rauscher's own summation of the issue was terse: "I would simply say that there is no compelling evidence that children who listen to classical music are going to have any improvement in cognitive abilities. It's really a myth, in my humble opinion." [8.7] On the other hand, there is almost universal agreement that if parents want to make their children smarter, they should encourage them to *make* music by learning an instrument. [8.8]

As is often the case, while we may not be able to prove the positive benefits of a particular type of noise, *i.e.*, classical music, we can and should be concerned about the *negative* effects that sound can have on a developing fetus. Nearly twenty years ago, long before widespread use of mobile devices, researchers were already raising concerns about the impact of high levels of sound on fetuses. According to a paper published in *Pediatrics* in 1997, a fetus first typically reacts to sound around the 24th week of pregnancy and do so consistently four weeks later, "indicating maturation of the auditory pathways of the central nervous system." The researchers found that exposure of a fetus to excessive levels of noise, typically because of the mother's employment, was linked to several negative effects, including high-frequency hearing loss, shortened gestation, and decreased birth weight. [8.9]

Some expecting moms work in environments in which the risk of excessive noise is obvious — those that work in and around aircraft, for instance, or in nightclubs, or in nursery schools, which you may or may not be surprised to learn are the tenth-noisiest workplaces. [8.10] But it turns out that it doesn't necessarily take high levels of sound to cause problems; even low levels of noise can disturb a fetus.

In May 2015, a fascinating study was conducted at the Wyckoff Heights Medical Center in New York City. Early research had already found that "resident physicians tend to have a higher-than-average rate of pregnancy complications, including premature birth, excessively high blood pressure (pre-eclampsia) and low birth weight." One common feature of their work is that they tend to carry communication devices such as phones and beepers on their hips for long stretches of time, with nothing between the devices and their skin but thin scrubs. [8.11]

Twenty-eight pregnant residents, all in their third trimester, agreed to undergo an ultrasound while researchers caused their phone or beeper to ring at specific intervals. "All of the fetuses (who were between 27 and 41 weeks of gestation) displayed startle response when exposed to a single generated sound. Responses included head-turning, mouth-opening or blinking, the study authors said." Some of the fetuses appeared to get used to the sound if it was repeated frequently over a short period of time (for instance, every five minutes); however, the startle reflex reappeared if the gap in the rings was extended to ten minutes. [8.12]

Dr. Boris Petrikovsky, one of the study's co-authors, made it clear that he and his colleagues were not blaming cellphones or beepers *per se* for the pregnancy challenges faced by resident physicians. However, they do believe that the noises generated by these devices can interfere with the fetus's environment. "So we now recommend that women not carry cellphones and beepers in close proximity to their baby," Petrikovsky said. "They should put it in their chest pocket or bag. The further away it is from the baby, the less chance the baby will be affected." [8.13]

That's Not a Hot Flash

There's a very good reason that medical professionals strongly recommend that pregnant women give up the use of hot tubs and saunas during the course of their pregnancy. A massive study of nearly 23,000 women conducted in the early 1990s concluded that women who had been exposed to excessive heat three or more times in the first 8 weeks of pregnancy had a significantly increased risk of giving birth to a fetus with neural tube defects, the most common of which is known as spina bifida. Of the common sources of excess heat, hot tubs created the greatest risk (a 3-fold increase), followed by saunas (2.8 times greater than normal), and to much lesser extent, high fever or the use of an electric blanket. [8.14]

The warnings about the potential impact of heat on a developing fetus are relevant to anyone who regularly uses a laptop computer. During the normal operation of a computer or any other electronic device, some of the electricity that makes the circuits function is converted to heat, which is emitted by the device. [8.15] Do a quick search online and you'll see hundreds of thousands of complaints and questions about what to do about an overheating laptop; such complaints are particularly common for those that have all-metal bodies, like the newer Macbooks or the late-model Dell that I'm using to write this book.

Most of the time, an adequately-vented laptop does not get nearly as hot as a sauna or a hot tub, so it poses a generally minor risk of harm to a fetus. Other mobile devices, such as smartphones and tablets, generally stay even cooler. However, there are circumstances under which any computer, including a laptop, can get startlingly hot. Running lots of processor-intensive programs, for instance, can cause any computer to heat up. One company ran a series of tests to compare the heat output of a high-end gaming computer and a space heater and found that they were roughly equiva0lent. [8.16] Another scenario, which is common when laptops are used while someone is lying in bed, is that the folds of the blanket block the laptop's cooling vents, which leads to overheating. A similar situation can arise through normal usage, if dust and lint builds up on the insides of the laptop, causing it to retain heat.

There are a couple of common sense precautions that can largely eliminate any heat risk arising out of the use of a laptop during pregnancy. First, avoid lying in bed or on a couch and resting the laptop on your belly, particularly if you are using a blanket or shawl. Instead, use the laptop on a desk or use a hard surface like a breakfast tray or lap desk (there are a host of reasonably priced options online. Alternatively, you can consider purchasing the "DefenderPad Laptop Radiation & Heat Shield," which promises to block "virtually 100% of harmful laptop radiation and greatly reduces heat emitted from the bottom of your laptop."

Radiation Does Not Differentiate

The fact that the DefenderPad lists laptop radiation as its first protective benefit is no accident. As University of Massachusetts Lowell physics professor Dr. Christopher S. Baird points out, every laptop computer emits a range of different types of radiation. These include:

- 400 to 800 THz electromagnetic radiation (light from the computer screen);
- 10 to 100 THz electromagnetic radiation (heat);
- 5 GHz or 2.4 GHz electromagnetic radiation (WiFi radio waves);
- 2.4 GHz electromagnetic radiation (Bluetooth);
- Low frequency electromagnetic radiation (emitted by electronic circuits); and
- Nuclear radiation including gamma rays (natural decay of elements used to build laptop). [8.17]

Dr. Baird, like so many others, is firmly of the opinion that none of these various types of radiation pose any threat to humans, either because they are inherently too low-energy or, in the case of the nuclear radiation, the quantities are so minute as to be inconsequential. However, that view is not universal. For instance, researchers at the University of Siena in Italy published a paper in 2012 that concluded that "Laptop is paradoxically an improper site for the use of a [laptop computer], which consequently should be renamed to not induce customers towards an improper use." The researchers found that the electromagnetic fields generated by various models of laptops exceeded certain international guidelines for women and fetuses, particularly when the laptop power supply was positioned close to the body. [8.18]

In 2014, a coalition of doctors, scientists, and non-profit organizations launched a publicity campaign called The BabySafe Project to educate pregnant women about the dangers of radiation from digital devices — laptops, cellphones, WiFi routers, *etc.* — and to urge them to limit their exposure. The group has ten specific recommendations that they urge pregnant women to implement:

- Avoid carrying your cell phone on your body (e.g. in a pocket or bra);

- Avoid holding any wireless device against your body when in use;
- Use your cell phone on speaker setting or with an "air tube" headset;
- Avoid using your wireless device in cars, trains or elevators;
- Avoid cordless phones, especially where you sleep;
- Whenever possible, connect to the Internet with wired cables;
- When using WiFi, connect only to download, then disconnect;
- Avoid prolonged or direct exposure to WiFi routers;
- Unplug your home WiFi router when not in use (e.g. at bedtime); and
- Sleep as far away from wireless utility meters (i.e. "smart" meters) as possible.

The group and its recommendations were quickly met with some skepticism. Over at HypeWatch, a blog run by the medical policy site MedPage Today, staff writer Sarah Wickline Wallan suggested that the claims of the group were inadequately grounded in actual science: "Without definitive science to back it up, words and phrases like 'damage,' 'behavioral disorders,' 'may lead to long-term health consequences,' are pretty hefty terms to be throwing around." In the end, she said, "[t]here is no doubt further research is warranted based on preliminary rodent studies that suggest potential harms. But likening cell phone use to asbestos and tobacco might be taking it a bit far for now." [8.19]

The BabySafe Project got a slightly warmer reception from the magazine *New Scientist,* which acknowledged that &lquo;if adverse effects were possible, the developing brain might be particularly vulnerable, as it is to toxic substances in the environment, such as lead." Author David Coggon noted that in 2000, a United Kingdom task force known as the Stewart Committee recommended that children should avoid unnecessary use of cellphones (a topic I'll return to later). [8.20]

The reality is that we simply do not know yet whether digital devices in general or cell phones in particular have a negative effect on the development of human fetuses. For obvious reasons, all of the laboratory tests to determine the effects of phone radiation have been conducted on animals, not humans. In 2011, for instance, Dr. Hugh S. Taylor, professor and chief of the Division of Reproductive Endocrinology and Infertility in the Department of Obstetrics, Gynecology & Reproductive Sciences at Yale University, and one of the founders of the BabySafe Project, co-authored a study that found that "behavioral problems in mice that resemble ADHD are caused by cell phone exposure in the womb. The rise in behavioral disorders in human children may be in part due to fetal cellular telephone irradiation exposure." [8.21]

If there is one thing we do know for sure, it is that huge numbers of people, including pregnant women, have adopted and are enthusiastically using cell phones and smartphones. Few seem particularly concerned about the fact that the sales of mobile devices has vastly outpaced scientific investigation into how those devices might be affecting our health. What that means, of course, is that we are all lab rats now.

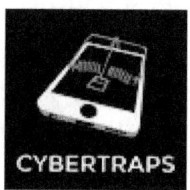

Chapter Nine
Your Little Bundle of Data

In many ways, bearing a child is one of the least private things a woman can do. A point arrives in virtually every pregnancy when it is obvious to everyone who sees you, either in person or online, that you are expecting a child. Unfortunately, far too many people are unwilling to leave it at mere observation, as one first-time mother complained on the subreddit BabyBumps:

> Never has my uterus or any part of the content of my pants been such a topic of general interest. I now realized I haven't appreciated the lack of intrusive questions about things that are normally considered too much info. Maybe I love secrecy, but I have my personal reasons that I really do not wish to explain to every person that wants to invade my privacy. Maybe my sensitivity to these questions is too strong, but let's try to turn this around: does anybody, ever, ask a man about the content of his pants, how his balls are doing, or ask when he will release something out of his genitals? No. Lucky bastards! I would like my uterus or the contents thereof to be a topic not open for discussion unless I open it. I don't want people to feel entitled to touch my stomach like it's content is public property. I almost I feel like I don't own my body anymore, it is now also my family's, SO family's plus the entitled nosy people of society who are too many for this to just be random unexplainable impoliteness. [9.1]

Her post sparked a lively discussion, with dozens of other women chiming in about the types of invasive comments and unwanted touching they endured during the course of their pregnancy. One particularly poignant post underscored the difficulty of an early unplanned pregnancy:

> As to the privacy thing… I can relate. Not as much NOW, but I got pregnant when I was still in high school. Talk about having your privacy invaded. Not only was everyone surely discussing me when I wasn't around, but yeah I was being constantly

touched and asked a bazillion questions. Ugh. [9.2]

The physical and verbal invasions of privacy that pregnant women experience are merely the tip of a vast data collection iceberg. As annoying as belly rubs and baby gender questions undoubtedly are (and I can only imagine how distasteful the unwelcome invasions of personal space must be), in reality they pale in comparison to the ongoing and deeply invasive corporate data collection and analysis that accompanies virtually every pregnancy.

A Cautionary Tale

As I wrote in _American Privacy_, personal privacy is not an object with a clearly fixed meaning, like a dog, a table, or a fruitcake. Instead, it is a concept that each one of us defines differently, depending on our own personal attitudes, experiences, and circumstances. And of course, our definition of privacy can shift over time in response to new developments, such as the invention of smartphones and the emergence of social media.

The "right to privacy" is best defined as "the ability to _control_ what information you share and with whom." If you want to share photos of your labor on social media, it is certainly your right to do so. The same is true if you decide not to share such photos. What people are describing when they talk about an "invasion of privacy" or a loss of the right to privacy is really a loss of control, the misappropriation and unauthorized use of their personal information. That's why, when Louis Brandeis and Samuel Warren first proposed a "right to privacy" in the _Harvard Law Review_ in 1890, they framed it as an extension of other well-recognized types of personal control: the right to prohibit trespass onto property, to be free from physical assault, or to recover for damage to reputation.

It's ironic, then, that given the fact that the "right to privacy" was essentially created in the United States (or at least recognized and codified), Americans have a more difficult time preventing the collection and spread of their personal information than many others in the world. That is particularly true for expecting moms and dads.

There are not many pieces of information more personal, private, and momentous than the news that you are expecting a child. For all of the reasons discussed earlier, control of how that news is shared with the world is important to expecting moms and dads. There are certain conventions to honor — telling family first, then close friends — and proprieties to observe, including consideration of the feelings of those less fortunate. And there are issues of strategy — when exactly do I let work know? A loss of control over the distribution of such momentous news is a significant invasion of personal privacy and under the wrong circumstances, can cause serious emotional, financial, and possibly physical harm.

The *ur*-story regarding a loss of pregnancy privacy was published in the *New York Times Magazine* in 2012 by Charles Duhigg. He wrote a lengthy essay on the new advances in consumer data mining and the sophisticated algorithms that were being developed to anticipate and shape consumer habits. One of the top priorities of these new algorithms is to identity female shoppers who might be pregnant, so that they can be targeted with advertising and coupons for pregnancy and birth-related items when they are statistically most likely to use them, in the second trimester of their pregnancy.

In one of the most commonly-cited anecdotes in his piece, Duhigg recounted the tale of an angry father who stormed into a Target store near Minneapolis and demanded to know why an advertising flyer filled with maternity products had been sent by name to his high school-aged daughter. As Duhigg explained in detail, Target has been a leader in the retail sector in collecting and analyzing customer data. The store manager apologized in person and a few days later, again on the phone. A somewhat embarrassed father admitted to the manager that the Target algorithm knew more than he had. "It turns out there's been some activities in my house I haven't been completely aware of. She's due in August. I owe you an apology." [9.3]

This is a classic example of an invasion of privacy and a precursor to where we are all headed: The unnamed young woman, who by now presumably is the mother of a 4-year-old, lost her ability to control the distribution of a very personal piece of information thanks to the relentless combination of consumer data, a computer algorithm, and direct mail advertising. It is not difficult to imagine circumstances in which that loss of control could have harsh consequences.

The Value of Pregnancy Data

So what drives Target and so many other companies to pursue ever more sophisticated data analysis to identify pregnant and soon-to-be pregnant women? The answer will come as a shock to no one: sex, or at least its logical by-product, sells.

Eleven cents. According to a study by *Financial Times* in 2013, that's how much advertisers were willing to pay per person for the identity and related data of pregnant women in their second trimester, the time when pregnancy and birth-related purchases begin to accelerate. It doesn't sound like that much, until you realize that the amount advertisers were willing to pay at the same time for members of the general public was just .0005 cents, or 1/220th the price of expecting moms. [9.4]

If there is one incontestable take-away for this book, it is that pregnancy is Big Business and every pregnant couple is a highly valuable advertising target. As we've seen, corporate interest starts at the very moment of conception or even beforehand, if you decide to start searching conception-related topics online. It basically continues until your child leaves for college. It's not unreasonable to think that in this day and age, there is very little that can be done about the rampant collection and analysis of data. In that respect, privacy is a little bit like the weather; as one wit once said, "Everyone complains about the weather, but nobody does anything about it. [9.5]

Of course, even if we can't stop the rain, that doesn't mean we have to get wet. It's not like people have stopped buying raincoats and umbrellas, after all. The same is true for expecting moms and dads. You may not be able to do anything about the market forces that make you such an attractive data mining target but you can try to make some informed choices about what data you share and with whom.

Whose Data Is It Anyway?

One of the first things that you should carefully consider, both individually and as a couple, is whether you want to share pregnancy-related information on a Web site or a mobile app. For expecting moms, it can be tempting to do so. The Web sites and apps offer convenient tools for tracking various pregnancy milestones, offer large amounts of information that may or may not be accurate, and typically have active forums and communities of other expecting or recently-delivered moms who can offer insights into their experiences. All of this can be very helpful to an expecting mom and her partner.

Thanks to the combination of a highly-motivated demographic and highly valuable consumer data, the pregnancy app marketplace is very, very crowded. Type in the word "pregnant" in the Apple iTunes store and a grid of over 80 of the top apps appears. There are hundreds more lurking in the various corners of the app stores. Not surprisingly, many of the top apps are published by well-known Web sites or authors: "Pregnancy and

Baby | What to Expect," "Glow Nurture," "Ovia Pregnancy Tracker and Baby Calendar," "BabyBump Pregnancy Pro with Baby Names," "WebMD Pregnancy," and so on.

The majority of these apps and their underlying Web sites are free, which should raise the obvious question: how are they paying for all of the server space, bandwidth, and software development? The obvious answer, of course, is that you actually are paying for the use of the app, through the collection and sale of your personal data to the advertisers that appear on both Web sites and on your mobile apps.

Free apps and Web sites that support themselves through advertising are not inherently evil, obviously. We all enjoy services that would be far more expensive or simply unavailable were it not for advertising. Well-known examples include broadcast television, relatively inexpensive magazines and newspapers, email services like Gmail or Hotmail, online file storage, and incredibly powerful social media. I use all of these types of services, so I'm definitely not here to reflexively trash the use of advertising as a revenue stream.

But alarm bells should go off when a company is collecting potentially sensitive medical information and/or the company does not have a clear privacy policy that explains exactly what may be done with the data. Those were the types of concerns that led the U.S. Senate Commerce Committee in 2013 to name 12 companies, including BabyBump.com, as the target of federal investigation into data brokers and their handling of sensitive data. At the end of the year, the Committee issued a report that was highly critical of the data broker/data mining industry as a whole. Committee chairman Senator Jay Rockefeller (D-W.V.) summarized some of the major concerns:

> [T]he data broker industry has been revolutionized in recent years by the tremendous advances in computing and data analysis. And as consumers spend more and more time socializing and shopping online, they are generating rich new streams of personal data to collect and analyze.
>
> These days, data brokers don't just know our address, our income level, and maybe our political affiliation. They have collected thousands of data points about each one of us.
>
> • They know if you have diabetes or suffer from depression;

- They know if you smoke cigarettes;
- They know your reading habits;
- They know how much you and your family members weigh;
- And they may even know how many whiskey drinks you have consumed in the last 30 days.

Like the pieces of a mosaic, data brokers combine data points like these into startlingly detailed and intimate profiles of American consumers. Under current laws, we have no right to see these pictures of ourselves that these companies have created. [9.6]

What we were only beginning to appreciate in 2013 are the myriad ways in which our devices are actively and often surreptitiously distributing our personal information. Since the introduction of the iPhone in 2007, there have been numerous articles about the amount of data collected, particularly that identifying your location, and the ease with which apps can access that data without your knowledge. As an article in ArsTechnica put it less than a year ago, "User data plundering by Android and iOS apps is as rampant as you suspected." [9.7]

Is an Off-the-Grid Pregnancy Even Possible?

It may be that you and your partner may not be terribly worried about the rampant data collection that is occurring nearly every minute of the day. For most people, the chief downside will be targeted advertisements that offer deals on things that you might actually need for your pregnancy. If the negative consequences are limited to such a minor level of intrusion, then you are fortunate.

But what if you don't want the targeted advertisements? What if you are worried that the information about your pregnancy might be misused in some more nefarious fashion? What if you are simply don't want personal information about your family and your medical condition added to the staggering heaps of data that is already being collected?

You could try, then, do what Janet Vertesi and her husband tried to do during her pregnancy in 2013-2014. Vertesi is an assistant professor of sociology at Princeton University, where she specializes in science and technology. She decided to conduct a personal experiment to answer the following question: "Could I go the entire nine months of my pregnancy without letting … companies know that I was expecting?"

Her starting place, of course, was to avoid any mention of her condition on social media, which also meant swearing friends and family to secrecy. No congratulatory posts, no tagged photos showing a baby bump, and no e-vites for a baby shower.

It also meant using her technical skills to change her browsing habits. When you conduct searches online or read various Web pages, that information can be collected and distributed to advertising networks. That helps explain why a search for a particular product will result in ads for that product and similar items on seemingly unrelated Web sites. For example, throughout the course of my research for this book, I've been seeing a lot of ads for pregnancy-related products when I visit various Web sites. To avoid having the same thing happen to her, Vertesi downloaded a program called Tor, which is designed to hide the identity and location of a user's activity on the Web. Among other things, she used it to look up baby names on BabyCenter.com without giving up personal information or browsing data.

When she and her husband made purchases for their baby's imminent arrival, they made sure to do so using cash only and did not use any loyalty cards or other trackable financial tool. "I even," Vertesi wrote, "set up an Amazon.com account tied to an email address hosted on a personal server, delivering to a locker, and paid with gift cards purchased with cash." Conspiracy theorists can make of this what they want, but there are even limits to the cash-only approach; one store used by her husband to purchase prepaid cash cards warned that it "reserves the right to limit the daily amount of prepaid card purchases and has an obligation to report excessive transactions to the authorities." Her efforts to truly protect her privacy during her pregnancy left Vertesi deeply unsettled:

> It was no joke that taken together, the things I had to do to evade marketing detection looked suspiciously like illicit activities. All I was trying to do was to fight for the right for a transaction to be just a transaction, not an excuse for a thousand little trackers to follow me around. But avoiding the big-data dragnet meant that I not only looked like a rude family member or an inconsiderate friend, but I also looked like a bad citizen. [9.8]

It's a fascinating experiment, one that brilliantly illustrates just how difficult it really is these days to actually control our personal privacy.

Without question, the most disturbing aspect is the revelation that the mere effort to control our personal information will be seen as a suspicious, even revolutionary act.

Pregnancy and Geolocation Privacy

There is one large category of personal data that Vertesi did not cover in her article: the geolocation information generated by her smartphone, which is collected, analyzed, and shared by a wide range of companies, often without the express permission of the smartphone user. It's a not-insignificant omission, given the powerful interest that advertisers and others have in your physical whereabouts.

Advertiser enthusiasm for geolocation information is based on two powerful concepts: efficiency and timing. One of the long-running goals of the advertising industry is to make the process of advertising more efficient. If a hardware store takes out an ad in the local newspaper or on the local television channel, its advertisement will be seen a large number of people who have no interest in the products offered by a hardware store. Retailers view that as a waste of money and would rather only advertise to people who are actually interested in the products they offer.

Until recently, it has been difficult to identify consumers with sufficient accuracy to make that level of targeted advertising possible. However, the vast collection of personal consumer data now makes it possible for advertisers to identify very narrow segments of consumers. That makes advertising more efficient, but there is still one piece missing: delivering an advertisement at the moment when it is most likely to be effective. That's where location comes in.

Every single cell phone, to one degree or another, knows where you are. In order to transmit your phone calls, for instance, the cellular company needs to know where you are so it knows which cell phone towers to use. Smartphones go way beyond that, however, because each is equipped with a Global Positioning System antenna that makes it possible to determine the location of the phone within a few feet. More recently, thanks to the rise of self-driving cars, the accuracy for GPS measurements is being improved to within a few centimeters. [9.9]

This degree of accuracy allows advertisers to make use of a technique called "geo-fencing" to target a consumer with advertisements that are linked to where he or she (or at least the phone) is at any given minute. The basic idea is that advertisers can use sophisticated software to draw a virtual fence around a particular location — for instance, a store, a city block, a tourist attraction, or an airport. Advertisers pay to use sophisticated software to track the movements of consumers that they think would be good targets for their ads; when the phone of a targeted consumer crosses the geo-fence, it triggers the delivery of an ad for that particular location.

It's one thing for advertisers and retailers to know that you are pregnant and to deliver advertisements to your browser or even the apps that you use. It is another level of data collection and analysis for them to know where you are at a specific moment. To be clear, the chances you will suffer any physical harm as a result of that data collection is quite small, although it can be a concern in domestic abuse situations. Nonetheless, some officials — including California Attorney General and current U.S. Senate candidate Kamala Harris — recommend that people turn off a smartphone's location tracker and only turn it on for short specific purposes, such as using Yelp to find a restaurant. [9.10]

You can find instructions on how to do so by simply searching online using the phrase "How do I turn off my [type of phone]'s location identifier?" That's not a complete solution, of course, since your cellular carrier will still know where you are and where you've been, but it will substantially cut down on the amount of location data you leak into the world. And if you don't want your cellular company to build a history of your movements, you can turn your phone off completely and only turn it on when you actually need to make a phone call.

The take-away from all of this is that protecting your privacy and the privacy of your family — *i.e.*, controlling the collection and use of your personal information — is very difficult today and is only going to grow steadily more challenging. As the t-shirt says, "You're not paranoid if they really are out to get you(r data)."

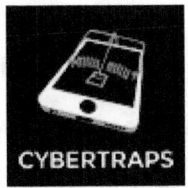

Chapter Ten

Social Media Cybertraps During Pregnancy

One of the trends on which I have focused throughout the course of my writing career is how social media facilitates the formation of specialized communities devoted to sharing information and providing support to its members — BDSM enthusiasts in Bible Belt cities, employees trying to understand (and sometimes evade) drug tests, homeschoolers, free speech advocates, privacy specialists, and victims of teacher abuse. Not surprisingly, some of the most enthusiastic and active online communities are those composed of expecting moms and dads.

There is good reason for this. Human reproduction remains a challenging, complicated endeavor. In earlier times, a pregnant woman would be more likely to be surrounded by a physical community of older women, family members, and neighbors who could offer advice and support. While some of that is still true today, the Internet and social media help fill the gaps that often occur in our physical communities.

As I said in the introduction, I am a fan of technology and a proselytizer for the benefits it can offer. However, I also have grave concerns about the overall weakness of data protection and the threats posed to personal privacy by that vulnerability. Inevitably, the intersection of information — particularly information as valuable as data about pregnant moms — and technology raises significant issues, particularly with respect to privacy and safety. Each couple should take the time to discuss their comfort level with sharing information online and understand the risks of doing so.

Personal Embarrassment and Global Ridicule

Let's start with the possibility that your baby bump photo might become the subject of unending public mockery. During the course of my research, I stumbled across the Web site Awkward Family Photos (actually, I think one of my sisters first tipped me to it). The site, which is an outgrowth of a blog started in 2009, specializes in publishing awkward or embarrassing family photos:

Childhood friends Mike and Doug began the blog in May 2009

after Mike saw an awkward vacation photo hung in his parents' house. Realizing there were probably plenty of other people out there with their own awkward family images, the two friends decided to create a friendly place where everyone could come together and share their uncomfortable family moments. Thus, Awkward Family Photos was born. The authors started by posting a few of their own childhood photos and those provided by friends, and the site quickly took off and became an Internet sensation; it now receives millions of hits daily and submissions from around the world.

One of the popular categories on the site, not surprisingly, are Pregnancy photos: women with a sonogram of their fetus painted on their stomach, bellies painted to look like fruits or soccer balls, a horse licking a large baby bump, a hunter who painted a target on his wife's baby belly, a disturbing photo of a man holding a baseball bat next to the baseball painted on his wife's belly, and so on. It's really quite an eye-opening gallery.

If you flip through the photos on the AFP site, you may find them humorous, slightly disturbing, or even downright horrifying. On the other hand, you may be inspired to create your special baby bump image to celebrate your impending arrival. Ultimately, that's your choice.

The single most important thing to keep in mind, as I have said repeatedly in this book, is that it is not possible to control what happens to information — text, images, video, you name it — once it has been placed on the Internet. You will never know if someone, somewhere has saved the image or has re-shared it. So that photo of the guy pretending to slam-dunk his wife's basketball-painted belly into a basketball hoop? Yeah, that's out there forever.

As Benjamin Franklin once pointed out, "Three may keep a secret, if two of them are dead." Just something to think about before you click "send."

Empathy Is Not a One-Time Thing

When you start researching "empathy" and "pregnancy," one of the topics near the top of the search results is the so-called "empathy belly." There are a couple of different meanings. Most commonly, it refers to the extra pounds that men often gain during the course of their partner's pregnancy. While it's not a particularly healthy way for men to cope with a pregnancy, it can lead to some pretty amusing photographs.

The term can also refer to a product created to help men appreciate how their partner feels at various stages of her pregnancy. The vest-like garment comes equipped with fake breasts and a waist level pouch that can be filled with weights up to 35 pounds, the typical additional weight a woman carries in her ninth month. There is even a BabyCenter.com video showing how you can create a do-it-yourself pregnancy belly using a reversed backpack and assorted weights. In a 2015 social experiment, three dads agreed to wear full-term empathy bellies for an entire month leading up to Mother's Day. They documented their experiences in an entertaining Web site: Three Pregnant Dads.

When it comes to the issue of empathy, we can all benefit from periodic attempts to put ourselves in other people's shoes (or bellies). In Chapter Seven, I discussed the fact that expecting moms and dads who use social media to help announce their pregnancy should be sensitive about the fact that some of their family and friends might be facing difficult reproductive challenges in their own lives. That is a concern that also should influence your social media decisions throughout the course of your pregnancy. The ongoing challenge that every couple faces during pregnancy and childbirth is to strike the right balance among the competing values of personal exuberance, efficient distribution of information, and consideration for the feelings of others.

Again, I am not arguing that expecting moms and dads should stay off social media altogether, nor am I suggesting that happy couples should never post pregnancy-related photos and videos. Social media is far too convenient a method for sharing family news and again, anyone who uses social media implicitly understands that they may see a photo or a status update that might upset them, often for reasons completely unknown to the person who made the post.

Still, couples should be mindful of their audience, and either create specifically tailored social media groups and lists to limit distribution and access, or consider sharing photos using methods other than social media. As I frequently suggest in my lectures to educators, parents, and students around the country, what we really need to do is to update the Golden Rule for the social media era:

"Post unto others as you would have them post unto you."

The Cybertraps of Baby Bump Photos

How the Bump Was Born

The stereotypical pregnancy update, the "baby bump" photo, is so ubiquitous these days that it is difficult to remember that women once went to great draped lengths to conceal their expanding bodies. But in August 2001, *Vanity Fair* upended cultural norms when it published a provocative Annie Leibowitz photograph on its cover: a side shot of then A-list actress Demi Moore posing nude, with one hand covering her breasts and the other cradling her belly, seven months pregnant with her daughter Scout. [10.1] Somewhat ironically, Scout Willis has grown up to be, among other things, an activist in the #FreetheNipple campaign, which protests bans on toplessness by women both in real life and on social media sites like Instagram. [10.2]

In the 25 years since that dramatic and culture-bending photo was published, dozens of other celebrity moms-in-waiting have also posed nude on national magazine covers: Cindy Crawford (*W Magazine*), Britney Spears (*Harper's Bazaar*), Halle Barry (*InStyle*), Brooke Shields (*Vogue*), Claudia Schiffer (*Vogue*), Nia Long (*Ebony*), Jessica Simpson (*Elle*), and so on. [10.3] Thanks to the enormous popularity of these covers, baby bump photos, both nude and clothed, have become a staple of mainstream and social media. A search for the term "baby bump" on Google News, for instance, recently turned up over 3 million hits; if you search Google as a whole, the number of hits climbs to nearly 16 million.

Without the rise of social media, our recently developed fascination with expanding uteruses would not have been that big a deal for the average expecting mom and dad. Not many of us are likely to be invited to appear on a national magazine cover. But if we have a Facebook or Instagram account, then we are effectively the publisher of our own national or international magazine. To varying degrees, our readers — otherwise known as our family, friends, and acquaintances — expect us to regularly post content that mimics the images posted by celebrities or celebrity-infatuated media like TMZ or *People*.

Depending on your personal sense of privacy, you may or may not be on board with the idea of sharing photos or videos of each month, week, or day of your pregnancy. Here's a typical pro-bump post:

> To each is their own but I don't see anything wrong with posting bump pictures. I don't feel like it's a private thing, it's obvious anyone can see our bellies now, and have heard of some people posting straight up breastfeeding pictures. That's a lot

too much for me but not the bump! I never show my skin though. [10.4]

On the other hand, despite working for one of the leading celebrity-bump obsessed publications, *Vogue* culture writer Patricia Garcia flatly declines to partake in the semi-obligatory social media sharing of baby bump photos:

> Now that I'm about four months along, I'm getting emails from aunts and text messages from friends asking, "Where are the bump pictures?!" Still others are scolding my photographer husband for failing to post a photo having to do with our future baby on Instagram. Neither of us has felt the need to blast our followers with our personal news. Other than telling our family and close circle of friends, we have adopted the attitude that anyone else who needs to know will eventually find out one way or another. [10.5]

It can be tough to swim against the cultural tide. If the paparazzi and tabloids are not publishing endless celebrity baby bump photos — a sample from just the past 7 days includes Keisha Knight-Pulliam, Blake Lively, Blac Chyna, Olivia Wilde, Kylie Jenner, and Candice Swanepoel — then celebrities are using Instagram and Twitter to self-promote their fecundity. But even in the cosseted world of high-profile celebrities, our societal obsession with baby bumps can be simply cruel, as Jennifer Aniston no doubt can attest.

The discussions over baby bump photos offer some fascinating insights into the fluid nature of the definition of privacy. For some expecting mothers, any baby bump post at all is a breach of privacy. For others, the photos are ok, but only if they are limited in number, shared with a small group of people, or don't show any skin. Still others draw the line at sonograms or pregnancy tests. All of these distinctions are an attempt to exert control over the spread of information but to paraphrase computer scientist John Gilmore, the Internet treats privacy as a defect and routes around it.

The Baby Bump Body Image Battles

It will not come as a shock to anyone who is paying the slightest bit of attention lately that people can be very judgmental about what they see and read on the Internet or social media. It is similarly well-known that people will post comments online that they would never say to someone's face.

Unfortunately, if you do decide to post photos of your steadily-growing baby belly, there is a significant likelihood that you will be judged by the size of your bump, your overall weight gain, your clothing choices, and even your choice of activities while pregnant. There is, of course, a term for all of this — "bump-shaming." — and a related Twitter hashtag — #dontbullythebump. All of this underscores the fact that when you post content online, you don't merely lose the ability to control who might use that information, but you also lay yourself open to whatever comments the world wants to throw at you. To be fair, many of them will be positive and encouraging and re-affirming. Far too many, however, will be mean, jealous, judgmental, or merely catty. You may have your own powerful reasons for posting photos of yourself online, but you need to have a pretty thick skin if you do so.

One recent example helps to illustrate the potential pitfalls. In the fall of 2015, model Chrissy Teigen and her husband John Legend announced that they were expecting their first child after undergoing in vitro fertilization. About a week later, Teigen posted a selfie on Instagram, dressed in a white sweater and black dress, showing a surprisingly prominent baby bump for 21 weeks; she captioned the photo "Somebody is early to the party [followed by 3 "no expression" emojis]." [10.6]

Teigen's post quick attracted thousands of comments and many of them were remarkably critical. Complete and total strangers questioned how far along she was, how much weight she had gained, and whether she might be carrying twins instead of a single fetus because of her IVF treatment. The number of negative comments was so high that Teigen initially said that she would not do any more "preg tweeting." [10.7] It didn't take long, however, for Teigen to reconsider her boycott; her Instagram feed has numerous photos that document the course of her pregnancy and show off her lovely daughter Luna, born in April 2016.

For Teigen, of course, posting photos to Intagram and Twitter that show moments from her life is part of maintaining her brand as a model and a celebrity. The fact that she has over 8 million followers on Instagram gives her significant social media "Klout" that has real economic value for her. As a result, Teigen has a powerful incentive to keep posting even when confronted with hostile, ignorant, or simply cruel comments.

For the vast majority of other expecting mothers, however, it is worthwhile to think about whether the your personal reasons for posting baby-bump photos to social media: pride, desire for affirmation, ongoing diary, *etc.* — outweigh the emotional energy required to overlook unwanted critiques and potentially dangerous medical advice. In an ideal world, body- and bump-shaming would not be part of the Internet experience, but that day may be long in coming.

In the meantime, if you do plan on posting baby-bump photos, you'll find some fierce defenders online. One of the most articulate responses to "bump-shaming" that I've seen was written by endurance athlete Brittany Aäe. During the course of her pregnancy, she posted an Instagram photo showing her baby bump side-by-side with that of plus-sized model Tess Holiday (@tessholiday), with the following message:

> in this image these two women are at about the same stage in their pregnancies - 39 weeks. that is the gorgeous @tessholliday looking boss on the left and me with the defined abs on the right. she is a voluptuous model and I am a sinewy mountain athlete. both of us are shamed for our size - she for her roundness and me for my smallness. both of us are having or had healthy pregnancies as validated by our healthcare providers. both of us are making empowered choices about our personal health. why does our society shame women whose bodies do not adhere to some narrow notion of false normalcy?
>
> let's instead keep our thoughts and words about other people's size to ourselves. pregnancy is tough enough without also being body shamed.
>
> #effyourbeautystandards #momshame [10.8]

You Are Now a Fetish Object

One of the more disturbing examples of how hard it is to control the use or misuse of publicly posted photos occurred last year, when several Australian non-profits warned that pregnancy bump photos were being stolen and uploaded to pornographic Web sites catering to those with a so-called "preggophilia" fetish (the actual technical term is *maiesiophilia* or *maieusophoria*). The circumstances of the case help illustrate the scope of the problem.

The story begins with the pregnancy of Meg Ireland, an Australian woman living near Sydney. Towards the end of her pregnancy, the petite Ireland posted a photo of her sizable belly bump on her Instagram account.

"The goal, Ireland said in an email, "was to reach out to my friends and family who wanted to see my growing bump. There were people on my Instagram who loved seeing my weekly bump updates - so I would post to keep them updated with how I was travelling. I didn't think anything of it, as a woman should be proud of her growing baby belly!" [10.9]

Somehow, an individual found Ireland's baby bump photo deep in her Instagram account. Using a copy of that photo, he or she posed as a pregnant woman to gain access to various closed Facebook communities devoted to multiple-birth pregnancies. The imposter then asked other members of the groups to share photos of their baby bumps, which he then copied and subsequently uploaded to one or more preggophilia Web sites. Ironically, Ireland herself was not a member of any multiple-birth groups; despite the dramatic size of her baby bump, she was just expecting a single child. [10.10]

A number of multiple birth associations in Australia, New Zealand, and Canada promptly issued warnings to their members about the incident and circulated the aliases that were used to create the fake Facebook accounts. However, given the ease with which new accounts can be created on social media, it was not clear what could be done to prevent similar attempts in the future.

Dr. Wendell Rosevear, O.A.M., who runs the Stonewall Medical Center in Windsor, Australia and who specializes in cases involving sex abuse victims and perpetrators, points out that mere sexual fantasy is not a crime:

> There are as many sexual diversities and appreciations and fantasies as there are people in the world and that's not an issue, unless one person doesn't respect another person's right to choice or privacy. Essential to valuing people is to respect their choice, so when you go outside respecting choice, it's called abuse. [10.11]

Dr. Rosevear's assessment is largely correct. While perhaps distasteful, the viewing your pregnancy photo online for the purpose of sexual gratification is not a crime. However, stealing your photograph and sharing it without your consent to others with similar interests is at the very least an invasion of your right to privacy. I'm not entirely sure that it qualifies as a form abuse. I suggested in a recent blog post that we should categorize the non-consensual sharing of intimate photos as "electronic sexual assault," but I'm not certain that the re-sharing of publicly-posted photos, even those posted with tight privacy restrictions, should be classified as a criminal act.

In any case, the real question is what decision you and your partner will make regarding the posting of baby-bump and other pregnancy-related photos. As I have said, there is no right answer here; it really just comes down to how comfortable you are with the idea that you really can't control what other people do with your photos once they've been posted. Meg Ireland offers a useful perspective:

> This experience has definitely made me more cautious about posting photos on social media. I don't share anywhere near half as what I did before. When I do post photos, I am very cautious about my surroundings, and make sure no one that doesn't know me in person, can figure out where me or my family is.

> My advice for other mothers would be to be very cautious about tagging your location in your posts, street signs that may be visible, and to be wary about what type of photos you post online. Children in their underwear should be a serious no-no. While it is nothing to us, it unfortunately can mean a lot more to someone with a fetish. Us mothers shouldn't have to worry about these things, but if you think of it now, save yourself the hurt and anger you will go through if they end up in the hands of the wrong person. [10.12]

The Cybertraps of Sonograms

One category of pregnancy-related images deserves some special attention. The sonogram has become a standard pregnancy procedure only in the last 30 years. The primary purpose of the ultrasound, of course, is to enable a physician to check the health of the fetus, assess its development, and look for any signs of abnormalities. But it is also a powerfully emotional moment for expecting moms and dads. When a couple first sees the splotchy black-and-white image of their soon-to-be child, a justifiable exuberance kicks in. Of course, something can still go wrong, but for the vast majority of pregnancies, the sonogram is the earliest concrete introduction to a new family member.

Hospitals have long provided couples with printouts of sonograms but today, of course, couples can take home multiple sonogram images and video on a USB flash drive, or have them delivered electronically straight to their inbox. That helps explain why there are tens, if not hundreds of thousands of sonograms floating around in cyberspace, on personal blogs, social media, and so on. If it can be digitized, it can be shared.

There are three main cybertraps to consider when thinking about posting a sonogram online: social media etiquette, misinformation, and privacy.

The etiquette question, which is an ongoing debate, centers around whether it is appropriate to post an image online that may show various internal organs, even if your healthy fetus is the star of the show. The anti-sonogram argument was summarized by one of the women who participated in a comment thread on the subject:

> I've always thought it was inappropriate to post ultrasound pics on FB. I think it's a very personal experience and I know I will not post it so that my FB friends (half of whom I haven't spoken to since highschool) can see. … I am 3 months pregnant right now and people already asked if I was going to post ultrasound pics and I said 'no way'! I don't care if I sound judgemental of those who do, it's just not me. And yes, I do think they are kinda gross when they are not mine! So far I have only shared the ultrasound pic with my sister and baby's grandparents, and honestly, I think that is all who need to see it. :) [10.13]

As you might expect, opinions ranged widely on this topic, from militant posters of pregnancy-related images — even going so far as to select a sonogram of their forthcoming child as their Facebook profile photo — to the truly reticent. Some had no problem with sonograms, but drew the line at pregnancy tests; others objected to belly photos too. Expecting moms and dads will need to make their own decision about when they cross the TMI threshold.

The cybertraps of misinformation and privacy are obviously more serious. Once it became possible to start sharing sonograms electronically, expecting moms and dads began soliciting not just "likes" from their online friends but what amounts to medical diagnoses. In 2014, a survey by the British parenting Web site Netmums.com found that one-third of all expecting moms and dads had uploaded a 12-week sonogram to social media to solicit assistance in determining the gender of their child. Some viewers try to guess the sex of the fetus by using the so-called "nub theory." The genitals of a fetus typically do not form until around 20 weeks, but in some 12-week ultrasounds, it is possible to see a small nub where the genitals will be. Practitioners of the "nub theory" claim that the sex of the fetus can be determined by the angle of the nub: If it points upward at 30 degrees or more, it's a boy; less than 30 degrees and it's a girl. Others claim that they predict gender by the shape of the skull and jaw displayed in the sonogram. [10.14]

According to Dr. Zhenya Pozharny, a clinical assistant professor at the NYU Langone Medical Center and a specialist in unique prenatal care, the idea of crowdsourcing your fetus's gender is "ridiculous:"

> Even well trained physicians and sonographers are often wrong using the "nub theory" I have been doing this for nine years. I always tell patients that I do not try to guess (because it's exactly that - guessing) gender in the first trimester.
>
> I am perpetually surprised that people do not view prenatal ultrasounds as medical tests. They arrive (frequently with an entourage) with an expectation of a "show" rather than a medical exam. One would never think to post pictures of one's liver ultrasound on social media. Yet pregnancy [ultrasound] pictures are everywhere. [10.15]

In the end, asking social media to determine the sex of your fetus is probably not terribly risky from a medical perspective. You hopefully will not make any life-altering decisions based on the uninformed opinion of your friends and unknown numbers of strangers. But I do think that it is inadvisable for expecting moms and dads to get into the habit of soliciting scientific or medical opinions from anyone who is not formally trained to provide them. Remember, the Internet can make you crazy. If you have concerns, raise them with your health care professional. If you feel the need, solicit a second opinion — but again, *from a trained medical professional.*

The privacy risks of sharing sonograms online are the most troubling cybertrap in this area. If you post a sonogram online, at the very least you are broadcasting the profile of the fetus's face, chest, and limbs, and often shadowy images of the mother's internal organs — most typically the placenta but occasionally others as well. But a surprising number of people share sonogram images that also have a variety of medical information printed on them, including the mother's name and date of birth, the location at which the sonogram was taken, the estimated age of the fetus, as well as settings for the sonogram machine.

Can any of this personal information be used to harm you or your family? The odds are exceedingly small. Nonetheless, the truthful answer is that you can't really know, because once you post the information online, you lose control of how it will be used. If it does not bother you or your partner to give random strangers access to the personal and medical information printed on a sonogram image, or if you conclude that the joy of sharing the profile of your fetus exceeds the minimal risk, then post away.

But expecting moms and dads should give serious thought to the fact that the publication of a sonogram image on social media is a violation of privacy for someone who is in no position to object: the as-yet-unborn fetus. The legal status of unborn children, of course, is the subject of fierce national debate; regardless of where you come down on that issue, most parents simply assume that they have the right to post photos of their children, both born and unborn, until they are old enough to object, which in my experience was somewhere around middle school.

From a strictly legal perspective, that is correct. Parents may legally post photos on social media without the child's consent until he or she turns 18. However, as I discuss in Chapter 13, the fact that we live in a social media-saturated world makes the right of self-identification and self-determination increasingly important. Sonograms, particularly those taken in later weeks or using the new 3-D/4-D technology, are fully capable of showing facial and body features. If the parents have chosen a name, the sonogram is frequently tagged with it. Already, an online identity is being forged, and expecting moms and dads should be sensitive to the future feelings of the developing person who will live with that identity.

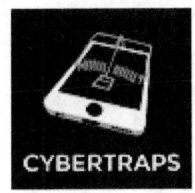

CYBERTRAPS

Section Three
The Cybertraps of Birthing and Infancy

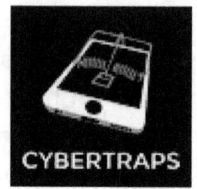

Chapter Eleven

The Cybertraps of Labor, Birth, and Birth Announcements

When my sons were born in the early to mid-1990s, the digital landscape was very different. Cell phones were still a rarity, and text messaging was in its infancy. The first message SMS was sent on December 3, 1992, just over six months before my eldest was born). [11.1] The World Wide Web was just beginning to worm its way into public consciousness and social media was nonexistent.

Those days, of course, are long gone. Today, any couple with a smartphone available during labor or delivery has the ability to provide family, friends, or even the entire world with a running commentary or even live video of the birthing process. If you and your partner have taken the time to sit down and draft a social media plan for your pregnancy (see Appendix A), then the odds of unpleasant surprises or unnecessary technology-based conflicts popping up during labor and delivery are greatly reduced. Of course, given the speed with which technology changes, it can be difficult to anticipate everything that new parents might face in the future.

Any couple who discussed and planned their social media activities before July 2016, for instance, would have had no way to anticipate the possibility that a bored partner might take a photo of a Pokémon Go Pidgey hovering above the bed where his wife was lying during labor. He was fortunate: His wife apparently just laughed and rolled her eyes. [11.2] Or who could have imagined that the game would spark its own "Awkward Pregnancy" moment? Giving new meaning to the phrase "long-suffering," one expecting mom allowed her husband to paint her belly like a big Pokéball to help entertain their young daughter. The video of the family playing Pokémon Go together is kind of adorable, really.

Not surprisingly, not every expecting mother finds the game play so amusing: Another dad-to-be shared a screen capture of the Pokémon Go character Charmander apparently sitting on the belly of his clearly irritated wife, who is resting in a chair with her shirt pulled up over her bra and fetal monitoring cables all over her torso. In a comment that may be

Exhibit 1 in future divorce proceedings, he wrote: "My boring wife is mad that I'm playing Pokémon. What else am I supposed to do to pass time in the #ER? DISCLAIMER: SHE'S 25 WEEKS PREGNANT, NOT FAT." [11.3]

But in general, as you can see in Appendix A, the technology and social media issues that a couple should discuss before going into labor are fairly easy to list. There is no single correct approach to any of these issues; couples can and should make their own decision about the level of technology and social media with which they are comfortable. But there are a few general principles to keep in mind:

First, if you share something on the Internet, you should simply assume that the information is now permanently available online and you have no practical control over how that information will be used or by whom.

Second, be mindful of the fact that while you and your wife may agree with each other to appear in photos and videos, that doesn't mean that everyone else in the room, including your newborn, has done so as well. At the very least, you should ask other adults if they are willing to appear in any photos or videos you take. Some hospitals may require that you get consent forms from the staff, a step you may want to take simply as a matter of course.

Third, birth is typically a messy process that by necessity involves the exposure of body parts that are normally not shown to the public. If your partner is planning to photograph or shoot video of you giving birth, or if you bravely are going to self-photograph, keep in mind that some of your photos may violate the terms of service for whichever social media platform you are using. We are only just getting to the point at which it is acceptable for women to share photos of themselves breastfeeding their babies, but most social media channels still draw a line at photos that explicitly show the crowning of an infant, even if you are so inclined as to share it in the first place.

There are, of course, myriad reasons why you might decide to share some or all of your labor and birthing experience online. How much you share and how broadly is a conversation that you will need to have as a couple. Again, keep in mind that once you share the information on the Internet in general or social media in particular, you lose the ability to control where that information will go and how it will be used. For the vast majority of people, nothing unpleasant or harmful will occur, but you and your partner will need to decide how much or how little you want the world to be part of your birthing process.

How Much Social Media Do You Want in the Delivery Room?

Texting, Messaging, and Tweeting

In February 2011, writer Tina Cassidy, author of _Birth: The Surprising Story of How We Are Born_, sparked a lively discussion online about the benefits of texting and other types of digital communication during labor and birth. Cassidy argued that the impulse to use texting and social media to share the process and outcome of birth is an unconscious effort to recreate the days when new mothers would be surrounded by older female relatives and neighbors during a home birth.

> These women intuitively knew that their mere presence helped the mother. In fact, studies have shown that mammals get a boost of the "love" hormone oxytocin when they feel protected by those they know, and oxytocin works to speed labor. The opposite happens when they are surrounded by strangers in white coats, which could be why many of those giving birth in a hospital wind up having their labors stall and needing doses of Pitocin, an artificial version of the same hormone, to restart their contractions. [11.4]

Needless to say, not everyone agreed with Cassidy's advocacy of social media birthing. Over at The Stir, an online magazine published by CafeMom.com, writer Jeanne Sagar asked her readers whether "birth should be a social experience?" Her own answer was a firm "no."

"My husband and I kept the birth to ourselves," she wrote. "It was us, the nurses, and my OB/GYN … and then, of course, our daughter. … This was the moment we forged our new family. It was only fitting that the people there were the members of that new family, and only those members." [11.5]

It's one thing to use messaging to stay in touch with family and close friends during labor and another thing entirely to share the progress of your labor with 333,000 of your closest Twitter followers. On April 5, 2014, Claire Díaz-Ortiz — an early Twitter hire and the person credited with being "the woman who got [Pope Benedict] on Twitter" [11.6] — sent out a tweet that read:

> "Currently googling: Did my water just break? #labor" [11.7]

The answer was apparently yes. Over the course of the next 12 hours, Díaz-Ortiz shared a series of widely-read tweets that chronicled her physical sensations —

> "Speed bumps on road and contractions don't mix. #inlabor"

her disrupted trip to the hospital —

> "Car now broken down. On side of road. Need taxi. #inlabor"

some family drama —

> "Husband upset he forgot his absurd ukelele to welcome child. In our broken car on side of highway? Prolly. #inlabor"

and finally, the good news:

> "Welcome to the world Lucía Paz Díaz-Ortiz! And to Twitter, @lucia;) We love you! #inlabor". [11.8]

Díaz-Ortiz's decision to live-tweet her birth may have been as much a promotion of her company's brand as much as anything else, but she's hardly the only woman or couple to offer complete strangers a social media window into the birthing process. A number of women, like Yorkshire resident Lindsey Thomas, have live-tweeted as a combination of social experiment and distraction during the tedium and pain of labor.

"I wanted to capture as much as I could, even during my contractions," Thomas told the *Daily Mail*. "It was a way of keeping my mind off the pain and telling friends what was happening. It was also a kind of social experiment to see what the reaction would be like." [11.9]

For one California couple, the decision to share their story on social media (again, on Twitter) was motivated by education and catharsis. In a long series of post-delivery tweets, Marco Rogers and Aniyia Williams recounted their dramatic and utterly unintentional home birth. What shines through this amazing story are their senses of humor and the potential power of Twitter as a storytelling medium. It's a great read. [11.10]

If you feel strongly about some aspect of your labor and birth, you can even use live broadcasting as an act of public advocacy. For example, when Ruth Fowler's labor started on Christmas Day in 2013, she and her then-husband, photojournalist Jared Iorio, decided to chronicle their home delivery on Instagram and Twitter in support of the practice of home birth. They used the hashtag #ruthshomebirth to make it easier for people to follow along. [11.11]

The photos and tweets that they published over the course of her 12-hour labor help illustrate the challenging, multi-faceted nature of personal privacy in our social media world and how permanent digital content can be. For starters, all of Fowler's tweets from nearly three years ago can still be viewed simply by typing her hashtag into the Twitter search bar and scrolling down to where Fowler first began tweeting on December 26, 2013, 8 hours after her labor started.

Her tweets range start out nervous: "Pretty relieved things are starting. Was beginning to think my body didn't work. Apparently all pregnant women think that #ruthshomebirth") She then progresses to the brutally honest: "1 more thing - no loss of mucus plug or breaking waters yet. Just - TMI! - diarrhea, which is a sign system is clearing out #ruthshomebirth" She concludes with her successful birth and painful aftermath: "Nye was occidental posterior and shoulder dystocia ripped me up! placenta wouldn't detach. Had to have blood transfusion #ruthshomebirth". Even though Fowler's Instagram account is now private, Twitter is filled with retweeted copies of a particularly intimate photo showing a completely naked Fowler cradling her new-born son on her breasts. It is a lovely photo but no amount of privacy setting tweaks will pull it back from the Web.

The fact that Fowler later chose to make her Instagram account private might suggest that the live-labor experience was not entirely positive, and that sadly seems to be true in her case. In a painful article entitled "How I Went from 'Poster Mother' to Pariah," Fowler detailed some of the challenges her family faced from the start, the fleeting nature of her Internet notoriety, and the dissolution of her marriage. It is definitely something of a cautionary tale for future social media birthers. [11.12]

Photos and Videos

For more than a quarter century, women had so much privacy in the delivery room that even their husbands weren't allowed to be present. From the 1930s to the late 1950s, the majority of America's expecting mothers gave birth in the sterile isolation of a surgery-like delivery room, surrounded by a small number of medical professionals. Over the course of the 1950s and 1960s, hospitals slowly began permitting husbands to join their wives in the labor room. By the 1970s, men finally gained access to the delivery room as well, where they could assist in the coaching of labor and share in the miraculous first moments of birth. It can be an intensely emotional and intimate moment for a couple to share.

Allowing men to participate more fully in the birthing process was a great thing for society as a whole and for families in particular. But the reality, of course, is that men and women have somewhat different levels of involvement when it comes to delivering a baby, and men often find themselves with time on their hands while waiting for the new arrival. Ironically, male boredom during labor is one of the reasons that we live today in such a camera-obsessed, social media-infused world.

In 1997, technology inventor Philippe Kahn was assisting his wife Sonia Lee in the birth of their daughter Sophie. Having survived the Lamaze classes, Kahn felt like he was prepared to assist in the whole birth coaching thing. His wife, apparently, disagreed.

"[T]he second time I said, 'Breathe!' Sonia said, 'Shut up!' So I said, 'OK, I'll sit at this desk and find something to do.'" Kahn's diversion turned out to be something quite remarkable.

At the time, Kahn was in the process of launching a cellphone software company called Starfish. In the bag he brought to the hospital, he had his computer, a digital camera, and a cellphone. Cell phones in 1997 had no cameras, so the only way to share a photo with family and friends electronically was to take a photo with the digital camera, transfer the photo to the computer, and then either email it to recipients or post it to a Web site and share the link. Kahn thought the process was unnecessarily complicated.

During his wife's labor, Kahn made a couple of quick trips to Radio Shack, pulled apart and rewired various components, and wrote some code to make everything work. By the time his daughter Sophie was born on June 11, Kahn was ready to snap a photo of her and share it with family and friends using his cell phone. It would be another three or four years before cameraphones would be widely available, but the adorable photo of a sleeping Sophie Kahn heralded a remarkable new chapter in human communication. [11.13]

In the twenty years or so since Kahn jury-rigged a cell phone camera, photography and video recording have become common delivery room activities. Nowadays, of course, new parents don't have to kludge together their own equipment: Smartphones today are capable of capturing every grimace, groan, and blistering expletive in high resolution or 30 frames per second. Even more remarkably, those images and videos can be shared with the entire world in an instant.

Not every hospital is thrilled with the ability of patients to record and broadcast what takes place in the delivery room. As the *New York Times* noted a few years ago, many hospitals have adopted policies that prohibit photography or video recording during a birth. One of the motivating factors, not surprisingly, is concern that photos or videos might show up later as evidence in a malpractice suit. A 2007 lawsuit for malpractice resulting in permanent shoulder injury of the baby, for instance, was settled for $2.3 million in part because of a video shot by the father. The recording showed a nurse midwife using excessive force during the birthing process. Hospitals also are concerned that the photography or video recording can interfere with the hospital staff or can invade their privacy. [11.14] These types of restrictions can be very upsetting to parents who want to preserve memories of this amazing moment, so if that is important to you, make sure you check out the hospital's media policy before it's too late.

Even if it is ok with your hospital if you take photographs or shoot video, there are a host of different issues for expecting moms & dads to discuss ahead of time. Understandably, many of these suggestions and recommendations are directed at soon-to-be dads, since they are not the ones actively trying to expel a new human from their uterus and thus are more likely to be the person taking photographs or shooting video.

- Above all, FOCUS. You may think that you are the reincarnation of Ansel Adams or Stanley Kubrick, but your primary obligation is to provide assistance and support to the mother of your child (assuming, of course, she wants you to do so).

- Have a conversation with your wife about the parameters of your photography and video recording BEFORE she goes into labor. The last thing a soon-to-be mom needs during labor — and there's a reason it is called "LABOR" — is to worry about whether particularly private bits are being displayed around the globe.

- Ask permission and/or get signed releases from hospital staff who might appear in your photographs or video. If you are planning on distributing photos or videos online, you should make sure that everyone present has consented to be part of your production.

- Unless you have made a conscious decision to broadcast the birth globally, spend some time figuring out how to distribute your images and videos to the smallest audience and with the best privacy protections possible.

- Consider hiring a professional videographer instead? The advantages are generally better quality photos and videos and less distraction for dad, who can then concentrate on assisting and coaching. The downsides, of course, are the introduction of a stranger to the delivery room and a slightly more crowded delivery space.

Above all else, don't be the guy who takes stupid selfies while his wife is in labor, like the guy who wore the "I Did This to You" t-shirt [11.15] or the guy beaming into the camera while his wife grimaces through a contraction in the background. [11.16] Yeah, don't be those guys.

Smile! You're on Facebook Live!

You are probably not familiar with the name "Ngangatulelei HeKelesi," but he may hold the distinction of being the first baby to be born live on Facebook. At just over three months old, little HeKelesi has no idea that he's something of a celebrity, but to date, over 400,000 people have watched the video of his birth. There are plenty of television producers who would be happy with that number of viewers.

As is so often the case with technology, HeKelesi is an unintentional Internet star. His dad, Californian comedian Kali Kanongata'a (who also goes by Fakamalo Kihe Eiki), apparently intended to record the birth so that he could share it later with relatives living in Tonga. At one point during his wife Sarah's delivery, however, Kanongata'a looked down and saw that his cousin in Tonga had posted a comment on Facebook: "Keep pushing."

Kanongata'a then noticed that his video had a rapidly-climbing viewer count, which meant that instead of simply recording his son's delivery, he accidentally was broadcasting it using Facebook Live. Kanongata'a told one news outlet that he did briefly consider turning off the video, but decided that it would be nice to share something so positive as a birth on Facebook. Clearly conscious of his audience, and presumably the Facebook terms of service, he made a point of keeping the video mostly PG (although there are a couple of brief flashes of nudity here and there, as you might expect in a video of a live birth). [11.17]

Presumably, Kanongata'a and Sarah discussed the idea of recording her labor, but it seems unlikely that they discussed the possibility that Sarah would give birth before a worldwide audience. Nonetheless, she apparently took the news in stride and dismissed the negative comments that some viewers left in response to the video. As Kanongata'a later told London's *Daily Mirror*:

> I know some people are mad that it's not private, but I'm from the island [of Tonga], and years ago, we would have water

births in public. I wasn't too worried about hiding anything because our culture has done this for thousands of years. [11.18]

While Tongans may have a long history of communal births, it is still fair to say that things have changed a bit. There is quite a difference between sharing your child's arrival with an intimate group of friends and neighbors who presumably are committed to your family's well-being. It's another thing altogether to share that intensely personal experience with tens of thousands of complete strangers. I don't think that there is a need to cast any judgment here; each couple can decide for itself whether the world is invited to the birth. But at the very least, make sure you understand how your technology works and do a couple of practice recordings to make sure that you are not accidentally broadcasting to the globe.

Birth Announcements

As I discussed with respect to social media pregnancy announcements in Chapter Seven, there are a variety of different issues to consider: Timing, family and friends, less fortunate friends or acquaintances, employment, etc. Many of those same considerations apply to birth announcements, but with one important distinction: There is a long tradition of formal, printed birth announcements that etiquette professionals suggest should take precedence over a social media post.

According to Cindy Post Senning, the co-director of the Emily Post Institute in Burlington, VT, there are a number of standard pieces of information that should be included in a birth announcement:

- Baby's Name and Gender (particularly if the name is ambiguous);
- Baby's Birth Date and Time;
- Names of the Baby's Parents and Siblings (include the full names of both parents, especially if the last names are different);
- Baby's Weight (commonly included);
- Baby's Length;
- Birth Location;
- Names of the Baby's Grandparents;
- Who Delivered the Baby (that is, whether it was a doctor or midwife, suggest Devra S. Renner, M.S.W., and Aviva K. Pflock, M.Ed. Psy, authors of Mommy Guilt); and
- A Baby Website, if any (with relevant information/photos of the

baby). [11.19]

Over time, social media has become an increasingly acceptable alternative for birth announcements. Typically, new parents include the same types of information that are included in printed announcements. As always, however, the important thing is to remember that there is a difference between information that has been printed and information that has been posted. The birth of a child is a momentous occasion and if possible, it should be announced with a formality that matches the significance of the event.

Of course, we do now live in a digital world and social media has dramatically expanded our social circles. You may have several hundred "friends" on Facebook, for instance, who have at least a passing interest in your life and the fact that you now have a new baby. Obviously, even the strictest manners maven would not insist that you send a printed announcement of your child's birth to everyone in your Facebook or Instagram feed. And here's a handy test of actual friendship: you know their home address. One nice compromise would be to send a printed announcement to close family and significant friends, and then post a photo of the printed announcement on social media.

Social media has introduced another not-so-hidden cybertrap: the adorable baby announcement competition. With only a little searching, you can find articles and links like these:

- "20 creative birth announcements that will break Instagram,"
- "Facebook Pregnancy Announcements" (over 1000 ideas)
- "10 adorable Instagram birth announcements," or
- "15 Creative Celebrity Baby Announcements."

And yes, some of them are genuinely adorable: the infant snoozing on a stack of baby books, or asleep on the front page from the day of his birth, or grinning up from a box half-covered with packing peanuts, or the one styled like a tiny mugshot for the charge of "Stealing His Parents' Hearts."

Really, many of the announcements are very clever and attractive. But in the quest for the perfect, not-only-will-my-family-love-it-but-it-could-go-viral birth announcement, it is far too easy to get sucked into an endless spiral of online comparisons, self-doubt, and competition. And your child's birth announcement is merely the first event in the online parenting competitions. It's basically endless and very little good can come of it, either emotionally or financially.

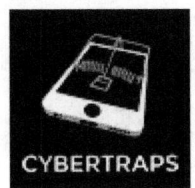

CYBERTRAPS

Chapter Twelve
Naming Your Child in the Digital Era

Over the course of a pregnancy, expecting moms and dads make a lot of decisions that will help to shape the course of their newborn child's life. Few are as momentous and long-lasting as choosing his or her name. A person's name is a significant aspect of identity over the course of his or her life. It can be a factor in a child's gender identity, interaction with peers, performance in school, choice of career, and to some extent, even future economic success. [12.1] For instance, studies have shown that the name at the top of resume can influence job interviews, call-backs, or even babysitting jobs. [12.2] It is, to put it mildly, a weighty decision.

There are a lot of different factors that go into choosing a newborn's name. A couple might have family traditions that are relevant, or a particular family member they would like to honor. For many couples, it is important to pick a name that has meaning within their religion. There may be a handful of names that you and your partner simply like and think would be appropriate, or you might find inspiration in the names of a favorite literary or television characters. The popular Web site NameBerry.com, for instance, reported that the name "Khaleesi," the clan honorific of "Game of Thrones" character Daenerys Targaryen, was the second-most searched term for girls in 2014. If you are technically-inclined, you might choose to name your child after an Instagram photo filter or your favorite little Pokémon Go monster.

Some parents establish a theme and only choose names that match the theme. One well-known example is major league pitcher Roger Clemens, who recorded the third-largest number of strikeouts in baseball history. He and his wife Debra gave each of their four sons a name beginning with letter "K": Koby, Kary, Kacy, and Kody ("K" is the baseball scorecard abbreviation for a strikeout). Boxer George Foreman took an even simpler approach: His five sons are named George, Jr.; George, III; George, IV; George, V; and George, VI. He also has 7 daughters, one of whom is named Georgetta.

Some couples choose child names that are personally significant to them as a couple. For instance, actor/director Ron Howard once admitted in an interview that he and his wife Cheryl gave their four children middle names that allude to where the children were conceived: Bryce Dallas Howard (the city), twins Jocelyn Carlyle and Paige Carlyle Howard (The Carlyle Hotel in Manhattan), and Reed Cross Howard (the street on which their Volvo was parked). No doubt the Howard kids were delighted that their dad shared that information with the world.

Should You Crowd-Source Your Baby's Name?

Perhaps you simply find the entire naming thing simply overwhelming. If that's the case, then you could think about the ultimate digital solution: Asking the faceless masses to help name your child.

On April 7, 2014, at 3:42 a.m., a baby girl was born to Canadians Alysha McLaughlin and her husband Stephen. They named their new daughter Amelia Savannah Joy McLaughlin, and shared with reporters an adorable photo of her just after birth, lying on a scale and weighing in at a solid 9 pounds, 3 ounces. [12.3] So what made her birth more newsworthy than the hundreds of other babies born in Canada that same day? In a word, her name — or more specifically, how her parents named her.

It turns out that Amelia's dad is a computer programmer, and in classic geek fashion, persuaded his wife to allow him to "crowdsource" the naming of their child by putting it to a vote on the Internet. McLaughlin set up a Web site, NameMyDaughter.com to solicit suggestions and accept votes from whomever visited the site. He then publicized the Web site to all of Reddit.com's users (2.49 million at the time) under the heading "IAmA Crazy man trying to let the Internet name my daughter… Yes my wife knows." [12.4]

On his Web site, McLaughlin made it clear that he and his wife were aware of some of the potential downsides to their approach:

> Hi, My name is Stephen and much to the disbelief of my wife, I have decided to let the internet name[*] my daughter.
>
> Yeah that is an asterisk, Unfortunately internet I know better than to trust you. We will ultimately be making the final decision, Alas my daughter shall not be named *WackyTaco692*. Sorry guys the wife wouldn't go for a free for all.

In a reply to a question from a fellow Reddit user, McLaughlin explained where the idea came from:

> I was sitting on the end of the bed after coming home from work and the idea hit me. I tend to be very forward person (this gets me in a lot of trouble lol) and I just blurted it out — 'Hunny, I am going to ask the internet what we should name our daughter!' She was supportive right from the start. I think at first she didn't think I was actually going to do it. But once the domain was registered she knew it was real.
>
> Hell, when I saw that namemydaughter.com was available I just knew that was the sign that I HAD to do it.

Although the vote totals are no longer on McLaughlin's Web site, news reports at the time said that the top vote-getter for the baby girl' first name was "Cthulhu," the name of H.P. Lovecraft's fictional and deeply malevolent cosmic entity. Apparently having no desire to spend vast amounts on therapy bills for their daughter, McLaughlin and his wife exercised their parental veto power and decided to go with the second vote-getter, Amelia.

Another option, if you can get past the somewhat cutesy name, is BellyBallot.com, a site that helps you organize a social media election so that all of your friends can vote on your top five baby name choices. The site also offers various prizes for the ballots with the most votes each week. It's a clever idea, but the site underscores the importance of paying close attention to the information being collected and how it is used. Like many sites on the Web, BabyBallot is advertising-supported, which means that it needs information about you and your visit for its advertisers. Here's a brief run-down of some of the information collected by BabyBallot:

- Collected at registration: Name, email, stage of pregnancy, and preferred gender for names;
- Optionally collected data to "enhance your profile": country of residence, home address, education, interests, birthday, baby shower date, and communications preferences;
- Collected from social media (Facebook or Twitter): access to you and your friends' names, pictures, genders, user Ids, connections and any content shared using an "Everyone" or similar privacy setting;
- Collected during use of the BabyBallot Web site: IP address, unique mobile device ID, browser and operating system data, time

zone, language, Internet service provider or wireless carrier, URL of previously-visited Web site, activity on BabyBallot Web site, and either general or specific geographic location (depending on settings) if BabyBallot is accessed with a mobile device.

According to the site's detailed Privacy Policy, all of that information may be shared, as needed, with service providers, service professionals, affiliated companies, to prevent fraud, with law enforcement, if the company is sold or merges with another, and with advertisers and advertising networks. If there is one good thing that can be said, it is that BabyBallot lays all of this out in surprisingly clear and readable prose in its Privacy Policy. Still, if that much data collection and sharing raises concerns for you, then you might want to skip the site's social media ballot approach.

Using Technology to Help Pick Your Child's Name

Hopefully, you won't need to ask your friends to elect a name for your child. But there are an endless number of inspirations for baby names, and given all of the competing considerations and the gravity of the choice, it's not surprising that expecting parents can get a little obsessive about searching for the perfect moniker for their little urchin. In pre-Internet days, the hunt for a baby name generated steady sales for shelves worth of books with titles like _The Complete Book of Baby Names_ or _100,000+ Baby Names: The Most Complete Baby Name Book_.

Nowadays, of course, technology can assist in the selection of infant names, with a huge number of Web sites and mobile apps specifically designed to assist parents in this important decision. Whatever your personal interests, beliefs, or aspirations for your child, an electronic resource is available to help you find or craft the perfect name. Whether your child ultimately agrees with your decision, of course, will take some time to sort out.

Among Web sites, there are a handful of options that really stand out. One particularly popular baby name site, not surprisingly, is run by the Office of the Chief Actuary for the United States Social Security Administration. The site, called simply Popular Baby Names, contains information drawn from every Social Security application since 1879. You can view the most popular names for every year, starting with 2015 (Noah and Emma), the change in popularity of a particular name since 2000, names that grew in popularity from 2014 to 2015 (Riaan and Alaia saw the biggest gains), and the most popular names in any state for any given year.

In 1993, for instance, when my eldest was born, the odds were very good that he would have one or more classmates named Tyler, Ryan, and Joshua. The Social Security site is a surprisingly entertaining look at trends in the nation's name choices. If it is important to you to find a less-common or even unique name for your child, Popular Baby Names will help.

Among the non-governmental options, the site NameBerry.com is probably the most well-known and comprehensive. The site, which is based on the work of long-time baby name experts Pamela Redmond Satran & Linda Rosenkrantz, is highly-polished and almost overwhelming in terms of the lists, tools, and articles it offers. Visitors can use some of its features to do basic searches about name information, but the more sophisticated tools require registering with a user name and password. The site collects some of the same data collected by BabyBallot (particularly IP address and so on), but is generally less invasive.

It is worth pointing out that the previously-mentioned BabyBallot.com does have a lot of information that can be accessed without providing the site with excessive amounts of personal information. One of the things that I found interesting is that the site offers curated lists of suggested names organized by ethnicity (ranging from Arabic to Yiddish) and by theme. Examples of the thematic lists include "Nature Names," "Heroic Names," "Tomboy Names," and "Rockstar Names."

Search Engines and Baby Names

As I said earlier in this chapter, there are a lot of different factors that come into play when expecting parents are picking a name for their child. I think it is a safe bet that w new parents are *primarily* motivated by the search results generated by their newborn's name. At the same time, however, it is not an insignificant consideration, particularly in the modern digital era.

It is virtually impossible to understate the importance of search engines to contemporary life. According to the most recent statistics, Google has 1.6 *billion* unique visitors each month; other search engines trail badly — Bing (400 million), Yahoo! Search (300 million), Ask.com (245 million), AOL Search (125 million) — but the numbers are still impressive. [12.5] More significantly, 93% of all online experiences begin with a search, and search is the **No. 1** driver of traffic to content sites. [12.6]

The simple reality these days is that when parents are considering different baby names, they almost certainly should spend some time testing the names and related nicknames in the leading search engines. Throughout the course of your child's life, people will be searching for his or her name for various reasons, including pre-date research, job interviews, background investigations, vetting for political office, *etc.* You may as well eliminate the more obvious problems now rather than later. Here are some of things that you might want to think about.

Unpleasant Associations

The most obvious question is whether the name that you are considering has any unpleasant or negative associations. For instance, if your last name is Manson, it probably makes sense to avoid naming your son "Charles"; similarly, if you are named Smith, you'd need a pretty compelling reason to name your daughter "Anna Nicole." It is unlikely that Orenthal James, or any similarly first-initialed combination, will be appealing to the many Simpson families, or Eric for the numerous families named Harris.

Beyond specific unwanted criminal and tabloid associations, you might want to see if a particular name is linked to a profession that you find distasteful. For example, as the *New York Times* reported, one couple decided to change the spelling of their daughter's name from "Kalia" to "Kaleya" after they did a couple of Google searches. It turned out that the first spelling is very popular with bikini and lingerie models, while the only other widely-known user of the latter spelling is a Goth graphic artist on the Web site DeviantArt.com. [12.7] You might also want to think carefully about naming your daughter Nikki, Angel, Candy, Amber, or Alexis; according to one industrious and overly-enthusiastic researcher, those are the most common names for adult film stars listed in the Interactive Adult Film Database. [12.8]

Unique or Anonymous?

As Kaleya's parents demonstrated, one of the ways to avoid possibly unpleasant associations is to change the spelling to something more unusual and therefore unique. Should you consider, for instance, naming your child "Jaxson" or "Rebekkah"?

The popularity and daily reliance on search engines raises an interesting issue for expecting moms and dads. Do you want your child to be a Googlewhack, which is defined as "a Google search query consisting of exactly two words without quotation marks, that returns exactly one hit"? Or, do you want to give your child a name that is much more common and thus not easily distinguishable from hundreds or thousands of other similar identifiers?

This is an important philosophical question for expecting moms and dads to discuss with each other. What are your hopes for your child? How do you see his or her life unfolding? Do you imagine a unique life for your child or do you envision relative anonymity as a better life path? Thanks to search engines, the name you select for your child will be a significant part of the answer to that question.

Of course, as the Scottish poet Robert Burns wrote in his poem, "To a Mouse," "The best laid schemes o' mice an' men / Gang aft a-gley." Whatever your hopes and prayers for your child, it's important to remember that their lives will unfold in unpredictable ways, thanks in no small part to the largely unforeseeable changes that technology will bring. In the end, it probably makes the most sense to choose a name that you believe is a good fit for your child, regardless of the search engine implications.

Reserving Your Baby's Digital Real Estate

According to the entertaining Web site HowManyofMe.com, there are an estimated 199 people in the United States named "Frederick Lane." Each person with that name has a separate identity and existence that distinguishes him from every other person with the same name, and other human beings are pretty good at telling us all apart.

But in the digital world, it is much more difficult to differentiate between people with the same names, and in certain instances, it can't be done at all. For instance, Web site names are governed by the Domain Name System, which only allows a single instance of a name for each top-level domain (*i.e.*, .com, .info, .org, *etc.*). So, for example, I registered "fredericklane.com" at some point in the early 2000s. Once I did that, no one else could set up a Web site using that exact same name.

This is not a huge revelation; most people have some experience with the fact that someone else with a similar name has already grabbed their preferred choice for domain name, email address, or social media account. But expecting moms and dads will want to think about whether their choice of baby name should be influenced by the availability of an account name in one or more of the following types of online services. In each instance, expecting moms and dads should expect that routine names are already in use; just be aware that the hunt for available domain names or social media accounts may lead to the type of baby name that will cause family eyebrows to shoot skyward.

Domain Names

If it is important to you that your child have his or her own domain name, there are a couple of different ways you can go about selecting a free name. The first is to start with a name you like and use a domain registrar search engine to determine if the site name is available. For instance, if you go to the domain registrar IWantMyName.com, you can type in a proposed URL and the site will show all of the possible variants that you can register.

If your first choice is not available, you can try different variations: add in a middle initial or the child's full middle name, use dashes or underlines to separate the words, replace words with initials, add in numbers or additional words, *etc.*

The other approach, of course, is to reverse-engineer the process and search for available domain names that you can use to name your baby. Not surprisingly, there are Web sites to assist you in doing this. One of the popular options is AwesomeBabyName.com, which uses the tag line "Find a Name for Your Baby that Isn't Taken."

The instructions for the specialized search engine are simple:

> Get unique baby name recommendations based on what firstnamelastname.com domains are available! Try your search multiple times for different results!

I put in my last name to see what I should name my mythical daughter and the top three recommendations were NavyaLane.com, JayleeLane.com, and SanviLane.com. Not exactly names that flow from my Irish/English family background, although farther down the list were MadilynnLane.com and ElanaLane.com, which are a better match. A second search offered up NathalieLane.com, MathildaLane.com, and PaytenLane.com. Here's an example of how other factors can play a role in name selection — as a New England Patriots fan, I can't imagine naming a child Payten, regardless of the spelling or gender.

All in all, it's an entertaining exercise, and if you don't have a specific name in mind, this might be a useful tool for generating some ideas. While the domain name system has been in place for over 30 years, the real stampede for domain names did not begin until the late 1990s, as the popularity of the World Wide Web exploded. You will find that over the last two decades, most familiar name combinations have already been registered, which is why AwesomeBabyName.com will offer up suggestions like Gracyn, Jazzlynn, Ximena, or Janiyah. Of course, if you have a less common last name, then you may find that you have a wider selection of traditional first names that can be used to create an available domain name for your future entrepreneur.

Email Accounts

The next category of digital real estate to consider for your forthcoming or recently born child is an email address on one of the three leading services: Gmail, Outlook, or Yahoo!. I can see the millennial eye-rolling even as I type that sentence. Isn't email dead, or nearly so? We don't read email. Only old fogies still use it. Yada, yada.

The fact is, email is a lot like Yogi Berra's favorite restaurant: "Nobody goes there anymore. It's too crowded." [12.9] As tech writer John Dvorak points out, people have been predicting the demise of email for more than twenty years, but nobody's come up with a replacement. Actually, that's not quite correct; hundreds of people have come up with replacements, but none seem likely to actually *replace* email any time soon. Despite its obvious flaws — the sheer volume of messages, the spam, the endless political donation requests, your crazy uncle's off-color jokes, *etc.* — email perseveres because it is a globally accepted form of communication, it is quick and efficient, it can be easily archived and searched, and it is asynchronous. Unlike texting and other forms of instant messaging, email doesn't necessarily demand your immediate and near-constant attention. As they get older, millennials and their younger Gen Z siblings will grow to appreciate that.

When my sons Benton and Peter were born, I created Gmail accounts for them. In 1993, I had no trouble reserving the name bentonlane@gmail.com, but when Peter was born in 1995, peterlane@gmail.com was long gone, which was no great surprise. However, I was able to reserve an account for him by simply adding his middle name: peterdavidlane@gmail.com. Both of the boys use their Gmail accounts for various purposes, although they've picked up other email addresses as they've gone through various schools and jobs.

I asked Ben for his thoughts about having a Gmail account reserved for him. His comments reflect a number of the different themes that I've discussed in this book, and may offer some guidance for expecting moms and dads:

I'd definitely say that when you set up the accounts, it was kinda disappointing, since this was my first real internet handle, and I wasn't allowed to come up with something cool for myself. But in hindsight, and especially now, it looks incredibly professional to have my real name, with no embellishments or substitutions, as my email address. I definitely appreciate it now.

As for it contributing to my online identity, I would say it does only to those whom I give it to, and those are usually family, close friends who I know in real life, and professional colleagues. I would say my Xbox Live handle is much more of an online identity, as it's also the handle I use on Reddit, which is most of my online commenting and communicating activity at this point. [12.10]

I think that Ben hit the nail on the head. I do think that parents can do their kids a favor by looking ahead and reserving a simple and rational sounding email address that can be used for college or job applications, or as a private email alternative to their work email when they are adults.

Social Media

This email anecdote also should help underscore the fact that kids start thinking about online identity at a very early age, and it matters a great deal to them. So, while you might think that you are doing them a favor by reserving a Facebook or Instagram account using some variation on firstnamelastname, or firstinitiallastname, the odds are even lower that they will thank you for it. One possible exception might be LinkedIn, which again is primarily used later in life for professional purposes. But for the type of social media that your child will want to use when they are legally old enough to do so, which generally is 13 and older, he will definitely want to choose his own username.

If you are dead set on reserving a name for your child on the most popular services, you can use a Web site like **Namechk.com** or **KnowEm.com** to check the availability of a particular user ID on dozens of different social media sites at the same time. These sites even check the leading top-level domains for you as well. For example, I entered one of the names suggested earlier by AwesomeBabyName.com — MadilynnLane — and discovered that I could reserve that username on virtually every major social media service, with the exception of Twitter. But what good does that do if 13-year-old Madilynn thinks that's a dorky username for Instagram or whatever the hot social media service might be in 2029?

It is difficult enough to anticipate or even imagine what username your child will find appropriate or funny a dozen or more years from now; it is even more difficult, if not impossible, to anticipate what the hot apps and services will be. Parents should do their best to pay attention to digital trends, because they are a significant part of parenting these days. But kids have an innate right to establish their own identity, both online and off, and parents should avoid co-opting that process as much as possible.

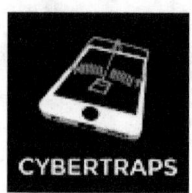

Chapter Thirteen
Whose Identity Is It Anyway?

The amount of time and energy devoted to selecting a child's name is understandable, given the significance of the choice and the long-lasting consequences that flow from it. When you think about it, few individual choices we make as parents extend so far into the future. Obviously, deciding to have a child in the first place is in that category, or perhaps insisting on support for a particular sports team, but there aren't very many other close contenders. The choice of a child's name is also the first opportunity for new parents to grapple with the idea that they are bringing into the world not the mere abstraction of a "child," but a new *person* with a unique identity.

"Identity," it turns out, is a surprisingly slippery concept. From the instant your child is born, a staggering array of innate, familial, economic, and social factors begin shaping his or her identity. Depending on the quality of your sonogram and your curiosity, the formation of your child's identity may have begun months before he or she was even born. Not only have you and your partner thought and talked about your imminent arrival in gender-specific terms, but you may have chosen clothes, toys, and even wall paint that reflect personal or societal assumptions about that gender.

Many other aspects of his or her identity are genetically predetermined and changeable only with difficulty: eye color, height, body shape, susceptibility to certain diseases, innate athleticism, and so on. Personality traits may also be tied to the specific structure of our DNA. We are merely at the dawn — at best — of fully understanding how our genetic architecture manifests itself in our psychology, our intellect, and our emotions.

That's the "nature" component of the classic debate. The nurturists argue, of course, that the more significant influences on our identity arise out of the environment in which we are raised: our nation, our state, our community, our economic circumstances, our family relationships, our name, our peer influences, and so on. Recent research suggests that the contributions of nature and nurture to identity are roughly fifty-fifty.

Regardless of on which side of the debate you fall, we can all agree that the concept of "identity" is increasingly complex and fluid. We can also agree, I hope, that each child is born with certain inalienable rights that should be respected. Obviously, children must wait until they are 18 before they can assert most of their legal rights, although I'll never forget one of our boys, then 4, asserting in a high-pitched voice, "But I have rights!!" Remarkably, he does not seem to be headed for law school.

Chief among a child's inalienable rights are self-determination and the formation of his or her unique identity. The challenge for expecting moms and dads is to give children the freedom to exercise those rights when we are encouraged to chronicle every moment of their young lives on social media.

Formation of Identity in the Social Media Era

The debate over how identity is formed and reshaped over the course of our lives was already intense enough prior to the introduction of social media; in the decade-plus since it has become widely available, social media has added yet another dimension to the issues surrounding identity. Unfortunately, the reality is that most parents routinely, even enthusiastically(!), co-opt the ability of their children to form their own online identity, chiefly by posting hundreds or even thousands of photos on social media.

Over the course of months and years, each photo gradually shapes a child's online identity in ways that might be quite different from what he or she would personally choose. Parents influence and establish their child's identity in multiple ways, from choosing photos that reflect well on the parents to selecting photos that capture the parents' own perception of the child: "Here's Mike clowning around again!" or "Tabitha's our little fashionista!" But when Tabitha grows up, she may decide to sing lead in an anti-hygiene grunge band; will the online identity constructed by her parents drive her to it? Therapists will get rich off questions like these.

Some parents will point out, correctly, that this type of implicit identity formation pre-dates social media and even the Internet. Of course that is true. The difference today, however, is that what happens online stays online. Without necessarily intending to do so, parents who post large numbers of photos and videos of their children online are creating a permanent pool of data that will make it that much more difficult for a child to establish his or her own identity.

The Importance of Modeling Respectful Behavior

We have four boys and as you might expect, each one uses social media differently. Interestingly, two of them choose to post much less frequently and for much more limited purposes. The other two tend to post more freely (sometimes too freely) and are more likely to use it as an extension of their real-world personalities. But within that group of four, one stands out as the fiercest defender of his online image. Some of the more intense arguments during his adolescence centered around whether his mother had any right whatsoever to post even the most innocuous photo of him on Facebook. There's more than a little irony in this, as we pointed out, since many of the photos that *he* has posted are the types of images that might raise eyebrows in college admissions offices. For a more detailed discussion of that aspect of parenting, check out the relevant sections of *Cybertraps for the Young*.

Nonetheless, there is no question that an individual has a moral right to refuse to allow the posting or tagging of their image on social media without consent. In fact, I think that few parents would disagree with the idea that a child in middle or high school has the right to demand the removal of a photo or post from social media if he or she doesn't like it.

The ethical question that arises for parents, however, is this: when does that right of self-determination first arise for children? Is it only when they are able to articulate their approval or objection? Or is it an innate human right that we should respect to the fullest extent possible from the moment they are born?

Obviously, a child's developmental stage does influence exactly how much self-determination they can exercise. For instance, infants have virtually no say about the clothing they wear or the food they eat. On the other hand, infants have no difficult determining for themselves exactly when they are hungry, tired, cranky, or need to go to the bathroom, as much as you might wish otherwise.

At surprisingly young ages, children find ways to demonstrate that they are unique individuals with their own preferences and desires — and that they have the right to change their mind. One day, pureed peas are the best thing on the planet; the next day, not even the sweetest cajoling can get the spoon past your infant's tight-lipped grimace. You quickly find out that he or she wants to crawl in *that* direction and *only* that directions. And much of the terrible twos can be summarized as a battle over the limits of a child's self-determination.

Depending on family dynamics, children quickly gain the ability to make their own choices on a steadily growing number of issues: clothes, books, games, television shows, friends, and so on. Of course, the painful reality, as most children eventually learn, is that there are some choices that are imposed upon them well into adolescence because it is in their best interests that parents do so — green vegetables, dentist visits, shots, school, chores, limitations on screen time, *etc.*

Social media posts, however, are not in that category. There is no compelling health or safety reason for posting about your child on social media and in fact, as we will see, exactly the opposite may be true. But even putting aside some of the Web's scarier stories, there is a simple and clear-cut reason to minimize the number of photos you post: modeling respectful behavior.

In early 2016, University of Washington researchers published one of the first studies to examine child attitudes regarding family technology use. The researchers had the innovative idea to ask kids aged 10-17 what rules they would like their parents to follow. According to lead researcher Alexis Hiniker, a UW doctoral student in Human Centered Design and Engineering, the answers fell into the following seven general categories:

> **Be present** — Children felt there should be no technology at all in certain situations, such as when a child is trying to talk to a parent
>
> **Child autonomy** — Parents should allow children to make their own decisions about technology use without interference
>
> **Moderate use** — Parents should use technology in moderation and in balance with other activities
>
> **Supervise children** — Parents should establish and enforce technology-related rules for children's own protection
>
> **Not while driving** — Parents should not text while driving or sitting at a traffic light
>
> **No hypocrisy** — Parents should practice what they preach, such as staying off the Internet at mealtimes
>
> **No oversharing** — Parents shouldn't share information online about their children without explicit permission [13.1]

Obviously, kids are a little conflicted about their desires; it's difficult to satisfy demands for autonomy and adult supervision at the same time. But the balance of child technology concerns are not dissimilar from the concerns that parents have regarding the ways kids use technology.

One theme that runs through many of the kids' answers is the desire for simple respect: listen to me when I'm talking, don't insult me by saying one thing and doing another, and honor my right to control my own information. Regardless of age, these are not unreasonable requests for any person to make in the digital era, particularly given the ways in which online information can be misused.

Some of the Risks of Sharing Child Photos Online

Before posting your child's photo on social media, here's a question to ask yourself: Would my child choose to take the risk that someone might misuse his or her image for their own purposes? Perhaps the answer depends on how the image is used. Unfortunately, because of the nature of digital technology, there are really no practical constraints on how posted images can be used. Unfortunately, legal constraints, such as copyright protections, can be difficult and expensive to enforce. Here are some examples of the ways your social media posts can be misused.

Viral Memes and Advertising

So let's see a show of hands: How many expecting moms and dads are comfortable with their child becoming the subject of global ridicule and mocking? How about serving as an uncompensated shill for Big Pharma? Thanks to the magic of digital imagery and widespread disregard for copyright law, all this and much, much more is readily achievable. Just post the kid's photo to social media and roll the dice. Here are a couple of stories that help illustrate what can go wrong.

As a starting place, it's important to understand the concept of a "meme." In typical Internet usage, the term refers to an image — preferably one that is amusing, provocative, disturbing, or ideally, a combination of all three — on which a funny or pithy comment has been written. People then share and re-share the edited images on social media sites like Facebook, Instagram, Reddit, *etc*. An image becomes a meme or "goes viral" when it has been re-shared by hundreds of thousands or even millions of people.

A well-known example is the Dos Equis "Most Interesting Man in the World," who unquestionably has hit meme status; search for that phrase in Google Images and you'll find hundreds of thousands of stock publicity images of the actor with edited versions of his catchphrase, "I don't always drink beer, but when I do …" Most of the edited catch phrases are, predictably, juvenile, indecent, and/or stupid.

There are numerous Web sites specifically designed to assist people in creating edited images that could become memes. All you have to do is upload a photo, from whatever source you like, and then type in some text. Of course, the same thing can be done using photo-editing software as well.

Photos of children, not surprisingly, are a particularly popular source of inspiration for these types of edited images. Type the term "child meme" into Google Images, and a disturbing gallery of child images will appear. Google even offers to sort the images into categories, the titles of which are disturbing in their own right: "Little Girl," "Death," "Kid," "Funny," *etc.* It is highly doubtful that many, if any, of the parents of the pictured kids gave permission for their images to be used in such mocking fashion.

Author Julia Fierro knows first-hand how it feels to discover that your child has become an unintentional Internet sensation. Two years ago, a friend posted an image on Fierro's Facebook page and asked the question no parent really wants to hear: "Isn't this your daughter?" The image showed a toddler scrunched up in a playground swing with her arms crossed, making a grumpy, beetle-browed expression at the camera. Across the top of the image was the slogan "Mood Swing." [13.2]

Fierro wrote an article for Huffington Post detailing her feelings as a parent upon learning her daughter's image had been misappropriated, the challenge and ultimately, the impossibility of tracking down and deleting all of the images, and the shock of discovering that the original source of the meme was a Facebook "friend."

As her husband later found out, one of his millennial-aged co-workers had copied the photo from the dad's Facebook feed and posted it to Reddit because he thought it was so cute. He later edited the photo to include the phrase "Mood Swing" after someone suggested the caption in a comment. Even today, if you type those words into the Google Images search bar, the photo of Fierro's daughter is in the top five search results. As Fierro acknowledges, her daughter's "grumpy" face may well be a permanent part of the Internet landscape.

> Our efforts to erase the photo from the Internet were in vain. As far as I can tell, it will live there forever. After a week or so of emailing back and forth with various meme sites, parenting magazine sites, and Reddit, we surrendered to the inevitability of the Internet. Surprisingly, once I accepted that the photo was out of my control, I felt better. Now, almost two years later, within the safety of retrospection, I even feel a bit of pride when I whip out my phone, search for "mood swing," and display a

funny and adorable photo of my daughter. It became a great
story to tell — Did I tell you about the time the photo of my
daughter went viral?

Not all misappropriate stories are so essentially harmless. Among the
"child meme" search results are phrases and suggestions that are highly
disturbing, concepts with which no reasonable parent would want their
child associated. And then there's commercial exploitation: What if your
child's image is attached to a cause or a product that you find profoundly
offensive?

That was the situation Canadian mom and blogger Christie Hoos faced
last summer, when she discovered that her daughter's photo was being
used without permission by a Swiss bio-tech company, Genoma. The
unauthorized use was bad enough, but how it was being used was
particularly painful. [13.3]

Hoos's daughter has Down Syndrome, and Hoos frequently writes
about the challenges and joys of her daughter's condition. But as Hoos
herself noted, "I never refer to my children by name, and rarely post
pictures of them. But once was all it took."

Some unknown person found her daughter's photo on Hoos's blog and
uploaded or sold it to a stock photo site. At some point, Genoma then
purchased or licensed the photo. The company made the daughter's photo
the centerpiece of an advertising campaign for its pre-natal testing product,
Tranquility. For Hoos, the implication was clear: her daughter was
intended to serve as a cautionary tale for parents who failed to test for
genetic issues during pregnancy.

Hoos and her husband contacted Genoma to protest the use of their
family photo and after some back-and-forth, got Genoma to agree not only
to stop using the photo but also to include some information regarding
Down Syndrome support groups with their testing product. Initially, the
stock photo Web site refused to communicate with Hoos, but with the
assistance of some "computer savvy strangers driven by no agenda of their
own, only a desire to right a wrong," the Down Syndrome page of the
stock photo site was shut down.

As Hoos understandably said, it is tempting when this type of thing
happens to just shut down all social media, and disengage from the
Internet. But misappropriation of images, particularly for commercial
purposes, is a violation of law. While there may be other excellent reasons
for parents to reconsider posting photos of their children online, avoidance

of digital theft should not be one of them; the burden should be on the rest of the world to behave in a lawful manner.

Given the realities of life online, however, and in particular, given the reality of just how easy it is to misappropriate images, expecting moms and dads will need to seriously discuss what level of risk and hassle they are willing to tolerate. The odds that a particular photo of a child will be misappropriated are quite low, but the headaches that will arise if it does happen are not trivial.

The Rise of Digital Kidnapping / #babyrp

Over the last couple of years, a new and slightly disconcerting trend has emerged on social media sites, particularly Facebook and Instagram: "digital kidnapping" or "baby role-playing" (the latter term is often abbreviated as #babyrp or some similar variation). The terms refer to the practice of social media users, most often tween girls, copying photos of other people's infants and children, uploading them to their own social media accounts, and pretending to be the child's parent.

The trend was identified in the fall of 2014, when *Fast Company* ran a story under the provocative title "The Creepiest New Corner Of Instagram: Role-Playing With Stolen Baby Photos." The piece described the experience of a woman named Jenny, who was startled one day to see a sudden spike in the number of her Instagram followers. That was followed by a couple of private messages that alerted her to the fact that another Instagram user named "Nikki" was posing as the mother of Jenny's infant daughter. "Nikki" had changed the young girl's gender, changed "his" name to Wyatt, reported that he was born prematurely, invented a birth weight and length, and so on. Once she created the new identity, "Nikki" responded to comments on her post as if she was the mother. [13.4]

For those who may be interested in the idea of #babyrp but who don't have time themselves to scour social media for likely digital children, there are even virtual "adoption agencies" that allow people to request children with certain features or characteristics. In some instances, there may be competitive bidding among #babyrp'ers for the perfect addition to their non-existent family. [13.5]

In general, the term #babyrp is probably more accurate than "digital kidnapping," since such impersonation does not cause any physical harm to the child. On the other hand, the invasion of privacy stemming from the unauthorized use of family photos, the inherent creep factor, and the potential emotional distress are all real and potentially significant. Initially, Instagram did not take the complaints of mothers like Jenny very seriously, but quickly concluded that such misappropriation and misuse is in fact a violation of the company's Terms of Service. Unfortunately, since social media accounts can be created so quickly and so easily, it is very difficult for even Instagram, let alone an concerned parent, to identify and take down every make-believe family. [13.6]

Sexual Fantasy

In some instances, not surprisingly, the harvesting of infant and child photos on social media has a darker purpose. As with pregnant women, there are individuals who have a sexual interest in young children. The condition is known as *pedophilia,* a term that technically refers to individuals who demonstrate primary or exclusive sexual attraction to prepubescent children. The term "pedophile" is often used to describe anyone who sexually assaults a child, but that usage is imprecise. Not everyone who sexually assaults a child is a pedophile, and not every pedophile commits assault.

What is incontrovertible is that the introduction of digital technology, combined with the Web and social media, has made it much easier for pedophiles to obtain images that feed their obsession. Last year, for instance, *The Telegraph* reported that a Russian photography Web site used by pedophiles was stocked with nude and semi-nude images of children that had been harvested from social media.

The site was reported to police by a concerned parent in Lancashire, England. The Lancashire Police issued a statement, however, that illustrates how difficult it can be to handle these types of issues:

> We are aware of a foreign website displaying photographs of children which have been downloaded from social media sites and we recognise that this has caused some concern.

> At this stage we are not aware of any indecent images and there are no concerns about the safeguarding of any children.

> This is not a Lancashire specific issue and as the website is based outside the UK is a national and international matter, however we are liaising with other agencies with a view to progressing our enquiries.

As there is an ongoing investigation into this matter we would encourage people not to try to access this site. [13.7]

Should you keep pictures of your children off social media because there is a chance that they are fueling the sexual fantasies of individuals in dark corners or dark basements around the world? That is only a question that you and your partner can answer, but during the course of your discussion, you certainly should take into account the current or future wishes of your child.

One English columnist attempted to put the real risk of harm in perspective. In 2013, Harry Wallop said, there were 5,547 assaults on primary school pupils. In that same year, there were roughly 8 million children in England under the age of 11, which means that .07 percent experienced some sort of physical harm from attack — the bulk of which, Wallop pointed out, were committed by someone the child knew beforehand.

> I genuinely do not have a problem if someone wants to take a picture of my child in his speedos as he does his lengths and later view those innocent pictures in a non-innocent way.
>
> Of course, I would be angry and upset, if the man (or woman) in question in any way approached, talked to or, heaven forbid, touched my child. But that's a completely different matter. …
>
> To treat the taking of surreptitious pictures, or the viewing of innocently-taken Facebook snaps, as some attack on a child is a gross insult on those children who have been genuinely assaulted. [13.8]

Wallop's position is obviously controversial, as the comments below his article clearly demonstrate. One person summed up the opposing view quite nicely:

> Wow, this is completely idiotic. Regardless of whether your child would currently know that they have been viewed as a sexual object before they've even hit puberty, they would likely know at some point in the future. It's your job as a parent to protect your child, and that includes from any future harm that might be caused from such a revelation. What kind of a parent are you to say that you don't mind if a stranger thinks of your naked child while touching himself? [13.9]

This is not a debate that is going to go away anytime soon, obviously, given the popularity of social media, parental enthusiasm for posting photos of their children, and the existence of pedophilia as a psychological condition. What is important is for expecting moms and dads to be aware of the potential risks and to make a conscious decision about whether the benefits of sharing via social media outweigh those risks.

Will Your Child Grow Up and Sue You?

If you are an avid poster of photos of your child on social media, you might want to rethink handing out a weekly allowance. Your child might be saving up to hire an attorney.

Sound far-fetched? Brace yourself: In March 2016, French lawyers and police departments began warning parents that they could face criminal penalties under France's strict personal privacy laws if they are convicted of publishing "intimate details of the private lives of others — including their children — without their consent." [13.10] The potential penalties include jail time of up to a year and fines as high as €45,000, or just under $50,000.

French attorney Eric Delcroix warned parents that "[i]n a few years, children could easily take their parents to court for publishing photos of them when they were younger." [13.11]

Delcroix's prediction was overly conservative, as is often the case with technology-related developments. Just as I was finishing this book, a report came out of the Carinthia region of Austria that an 18-year-old woman has filed suit against her parents for posting embarrassing photographs of her on Facebook. The woman alleges that the photos, which include shots of her having her diaper changed, lying naked in her crib, or learning to use the potty, have made her life miserable. She reportedly asked her parents to remove the photos; when they refused to do so, she decided to sue. Her father reportedly believes that since he took the photos, he has the right to publish them. Austrian legal expert Michael Rami told a local publication that if the daughter can show that she has been deprived of a right to a private life, her parents may in fact be liable for damages for pain and suffering, as well as the daughter's legal costs. [13.12]

Lawsuits by children against their parents for invasion of privacy are unlikely to become very numerous, if for no other reasons the expense of litigation and the difficulty of proving and quantifying harm. Regardless of how infuriating it may be to an outraged adolescent that his mother has posted a childhood photo from his tutu-wearing phase on Facebook, is the psychological or social damage something on which we can actually put a price? Aggressive lawyers may try to do so, of course, but I doubt in any great numbers.

Still, it is important to understand that there is growing support for greater individual control over online images or posts. Two years ago, the European Court of Justice (ECJ), the top court in the European Union, ruled that individuals have a "right to be forgotten." The decision came in a lawsuit by a Spanish man against Google, arguing that a search result link to the forced auction of his home sixteen years earlier was an infringement on his right to privacy.

The ECJ agreed, concluding that indefinite access to every aspect of a person's life runs contrary to data protection principles established by the European Union. The court ruled that personal data must be stripped from search engines when the information "appear[s] to be inadequate, irrelevant or no longer relevant, or excessive in relation to the purpose for which they were processed and in the light of the time that has elapsed." [13.13]

Needless to say, there is considerable debate about exactly how the court's ruling should be implemented. What makes a particular piece of information "irrelevant" or "inadequate"? How much time must elapse before something should be hidden from search results? Those are all tricky questions that will require a significant amount of litigation to sort out.

In the meantime, activists are focusing on providing children greater privacy protections before they become adults. In 2015, under the leadership of Baroness Beeban Tania Kidron, the United Kingdom Safer Internet Center launched a new initiative called "iRights." In the program's initial press release, Baroness Kidron explained the objectives:

> iRights is a civil society initiative that seeks to make the digital world a more transparent and empowering place for children and young people (under 18) by delivering a universal framework of digital rights, in order that young people are able to access digital technologies creatively, knowledgeably and fearlessly.

The organization has identified five principles designed to "interweave to tackle the multiple issues of digital engagement":

- **The Right to REMOVE**: Every child and young person should have the right to easily edit or delete all content they have created;

- **The Right to KNOW**: Children and young people have the right to know who is holding or profiting from their information, what their information is being used for and whether it is being copied, sold or traded;

- **The Right to SAFETY AND SUPPORT**: Children and young people should be confident that they will be protected from illegal practices and supported if confronted by troubling or upsetting scenarios online;

- **The Right to INFORMED AND CONSCIOUS CHOICES**: Children and young people should be empowered to reach into creative places online, but at the same time have the capacity and support to easily disengage; and

- **THE Right to DIGITAL LITERACY**: To access the knowledge that the Internet can deliver, children and young people need to be taught the skills to use, create and critique digital technologies, and given the tools to negotiate changing social norms. [13.14]

If a child is not old enough to provide "informed and conscious choices" regarding his or her presence and depiction on social media, then it is fair to ask whether *any* image should be posted online of him or her, even with the best of privacy protections. When parents post photos of their children online, they generally do so with the best of intentions: to show their parental pride, to introduce their child, to promote and maintain familial relationships, and so on. Those are all legitimate motivations but nonetheless, it is a classic non-consensual act to post content online of a child who is too young to understand the implications and consciously express his or her desires.

Many parents will correctly point out, as I said earlier, that they make a lot of non-consensual choices for their children during various ages and stages when they are unable to make safe, healthy, and rational choices for themselves. But it is one thing to choose an outfit for your one-year-old to wear — which no one will remember the following week, let alone months or years later — and another thing altogether to create a permanent, global record of that choice by posting a photo online.

Suggestions to Minimize the Risk of Misuse

It may well be, after discussing these issues, that you and your partner decide that the chances of someone misusing photos of *your* child, given the millions of child photos that are posted online every week, are quite small. That is a rational conclusion to reach. However, if you are truly concerned about the potential misuse of images of your child, there is one and only one solution: Travel frequently to visit family and friends so that they can see their new family member in person, and forbid any posting of photos of your child to social media — period, full stop.

This may seem like an extreme position and it can be difficult and time-consuming to enforce. It's also impractical, anti-social, and ultimately pretty anti-familial as well. Photographs and videos have been an important part of family histories and storytelling for the better part of a century, and it would be a real shame for fear to overwhelm our preservation of family memories and our sharing of happy moments in our lives. So let's assume that you're not going to go completely cold turkey on the posting of photos of your child. What are your options for minimizing the risk of misappropriation and misuse?

Before we talk about the distribution options, it is worth pointing out that absent prior agreement and honorable behavior, there is no way to guarantee that a photo of your child will not wind up online. You can, of course, try to make it slightly harder by only sharing printouts of photos or actual postcards with friends and family members. But if any of them have a digital camera, a scanner, or even a smartphone, a physical photograph can be converted into a digital image and posted online in mere minutes. Just think of the number of early-20th century photos that are circulated on Facebook, particularly on Mother's or Father's Day.

Assuming you trust your relatives and friends not to re-post to social media, there are certainly several options for sharing photographs of your child. For instance, you can buy a bunch of inexpensive 1 GB USB drives for about $2 each. A 1 GB USB drive can hold approximately 200 high-quality photos of your lovely child, which is probably more than even the most loving family member will want to flip through in a single setting. Send out a USB stick to grandparents, siblings, and close friends every 3-4 months with a firm request that the photos stay on the drive.

If you prefer electronic solutions, the easiest is to create a **.zip** file of your favorite photos and send it to family and friends by email. Keep in mind, of course, that less tech-savvy recipients might not be comfortable with the technical steps necessary to unzip an attachment and view the uncompressed photos. A slightly easier digital approach is to upload photos of your new arrival to one of the numerous online storage sites like Dropbox, Google Drive, Box, OneDrive, IDrive, or SugarSync. Most if not all offer you the ability to share a specific folder or album with one or more people. Once you've set up your folder and invited family and friends to share it, they can see whatever photos or videos you put in it.

However, if you and your partner still want to enjoy the advantages of social media — rapid distribution, efficient spread of information, effective communication with a far-flung family, nearly-instantaneous and communal feedback — then there are steps you can take to minimize the risk of unauthorized downloading and use of your child's photo. Given how frequently social media sites change their privacy controls, and given the rapidity with which new social media sites pop up, it's really not possible to provide specific instructions. My best recommendation, if you and your partner are discussing this issue, is to do an online search for a phrase similar to "protect child photos online." Any of the leading search engines will provide links to the latest recommendations on parenting and digital safety sites. Here are some general principles to keep in mind:

- Make use of albums and groups, use the tightest privacy settings possible, and be thoughtful about who you include in the group.
- Talk to each person in the group about your family's privacy expectations and stress how important it is that they not re-share photos without permission.
- Consider using software to put a watermark on your shared photos, which would reduce the likelihood of unauthorized use for commercial advertising.
- Reduce the resolution of your photos before you post them; the lower the resolution, the less likely it is that a particular photo will be stolen, particularly for advertising.
- Turn off location services when using your smartphone to take or upload photos.
- If you don't want to broadcast the location in which your child was photographed, avoid using well-known locations or landmarks as backdrops.
- Remember the Golden Rule of Social Media: "Post unto others as you would have them post unto you." Don't upload photos of someone else's child without the consent of their parents (and if the child is old enough, the child as well). [13.15]

It is worth reiterating that the chances your child will suffer any physical harm if you share photos on social media is *exceedingly* small. However, the chances of one or more photos being used in a way that makes you uncomfortable or of which you would not approve is not negligible. You and your partner will need to decide the level of sharing with which you are both comfortable.

What is certain, however, is that every photo you choose to post of your newborn limits, however slightly, her ability to establish her own unique identity in the future, both online and to a certain extent, off-line as well. Think carefully about your reasons for posting photos of your child online and ask yourself whether your child's inherent rights of identity and self-determination should outweigh them.

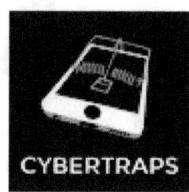

Chapter Fourteen

"Smart Technology" for New Parents

So here's a quick test of just how much you love technology and data and/or how freaked out you are about becoming parents: Are you willing to plunk down $249 for a medium-tech changing pad? The product in question is called the "Hatch Baby," a changing pad that comes with a built-in scale and a companion smartphone app which together are designed to track a range of information about your new baby, including:

- Your baby's weight gain;
- The amount your baby eats at each feeding;
- The weight of your baby's wet or messy diapers;
- The length of your baby; and
- The amount of time your baby sleeps.

As a recent article in *Time* put it, "Today's newborns could be the first generation to be tracked from birth." It will be years if not decades before we will fully understand the implications of cradle-to-grave observation and surveillance. The question is just how much you and your partner want to contribute to this trend and how easily you can opt out. As we'll see in the next chapter, there is a legitimate concern that you might get so caught in the quantifying of your newborn's life that you overlook the sheer joy of your baby's first days, weeks, and months.

Whatever your natural inclinations, be prepared: Manufacturers and retailers will do their absolute best to convince you that unless you purchase the absolute latest in "smart" infant gear, all kinds of terrible things will happen. To the best of your ability, resist the sales pitches. You may be raising a digital native, but you don't have to digitally record every instant of your child's life.

IoBT (the Internet of Baby Things)

Tech Invades the Nursery

The Hatch Baby and other products like it are part of a growing wave of so-called "smart" devices and apps that are being targeted at an increasingly tech-savvy generation of expecting moms and dads. The appeal is obvious: Notwithstanding the _Brave New World_ overtones of its name, the company's marketing is based on a simple premise: who wouldn't want the reassurance of collected and analyzed data that can track a child's healthy development? Hatch Baby offers assurance or warnings of potential problems by comparing each baby's "growth percentile to worldwide (World Health Organization) data and Hatch babies like yours."

Needless to say, though, there are a couple of significant issues that parents should consider before plunking down that kind of money on Hatch Baby or any other "smart" baby equipment: 1) What are the privacy implications; and 2) Will you actually use it?

Let's start with the practical consideration. You and your partner will want to have a frank and realistic conversation about just how diligent you each will be about actually using your expensive new changing table to collect and record data in the first place. A reviewer for the tech Web site c|net neatly summarized the issue:

> The problem, as I mentioned before, comes with the actual data collection. It's not only during movies [when parents may choose to change their infant on the couch rather than stop the movie] — when you're waking up in the middle of the night, the last thing you want to do is pull out your phone to record the number of ounces your kid just ate. You can go back to add entries, but I quickly ran into the problem of partial or estimated data. That meant Hatch Baby didn't demystify my son's schedule any more than just living with him. [14.1]

Let's be clear: I love technology and I have periodically used a variety of electronic documents and apps to track a wide range of personal data, including words written per day, running mileage, daily glasses of water, steps, weight [ugh!], _etc._. My intent is virtuous, but various distractions inevitably create holes in both the recording of data and my resolve. With disturbing rapidity, the value of the recorded data diminishes and the point of the entire exercise vanishes.

There's one other minor detail to point out. The changing pad itself requires four C batteries in order for the scale to function. Although I've never used the Hatch Baby, more than half a century of life experience qualifies me to predict that the batteries inevitably will need replacing at 2 a.m. one night, when you are dealing with your third messy diaper of the evening and your fourteenth night in a row with no more than 3 consecutive hours of sleep. Even if you are foresighted enough to have spare C batteries somewhere in your house, it is a safe bet that you will choose a swift return to bed over fumbling through kitchen drawers or a tool box in the garage looking for replacements.

Obviously, there are some circumstances in which this product could be useful. If your child has a medical condition that requires that level of dedication and attention to detail, you will undoubtedly be grateful for the data collection and analysis the Hatch Baby provides, and you will probably be organized enough to keep the necessary batteries nearby. But I suspect that for the vast majority of parents, this technology is more labor-intensive and habit-demanding than "smart."

The privacy implications are obvious and of greater concern. Every bit of data that you enter into the app, "including, but not limited to, child's weight, child's feeding amount, child's sleep, etc.," is collected, stored, and analyzed by Hatch Baby. The company promises that it "will never sell your Personally Identifiable Information [PII], but we may sell aggregated, anonymized forms of information to third parties."

Unfortunately, it is increasingly evident that "anonymized" data is anything but. In a post to help celebrate "Choose Privacy Week 2015," the American Library Association pointed out that even after PII has been removed from collected data, individuals can still be identified.

> Recent experiments have shown, in some cases unintentionally, the surprising ease with which apparently anonymous data can be "reidentified,' that is, combined in a manner that results in identifying individuals to a great degree of certainty." [14.2]

The important thing to keep in mind is that anonymized data is of greatest value to government planners and sociologists, who deal in broad public trends. Individuals and companies that are looking to sell things, on the other hand, are much more interested in de-anonymized data, since that enables them to better target their advertising to interested consumers, which ideally will lead to greater sales. The whistle-blowing informant Deep Throat, a key figure in the epic Watergate scandal chronicled in _All the President's Men_ was right: "Follow the money."

It may be that you are not terribly concerned about this type of privacy issue, or you see the value of the data analysis by Hatch Baby as a fair exchange for the collected information. That's a perfectly reasonable conclusion for you and your partner to reach, of course, when you use services that collect and supposedly anonymize your own data. But you should think about whether you have an obligation to be even more careful with your child's data, until such time as he or she can begin participating in discussions about what data to share and with whom.

Another company that is attracting media attention for its "smart" baby technology is Mimo, which markets a real-time breathing and sleep monitoring system. The Mimo system has several components: cotton pajamas with various washable sensors sewn in, a small pod (called a "turtle") that snaps onto the pajamas to collect data from the sensors and transmit it to a nearby base (called a "lilypad") for uploading to the cloud, and a smartphone app for downloading and displaying the analyzed data. Here's the company's own product description:

> The Mimo Smart Baby Monitor uses all-cotton kimonos and bodysuits to show you your baby's breathing, sleeping temperature, body position, activity level, and whether they are awake and asleep, all right to your smartphone. Using Bluetooth Low Energy (the safest technology available), this information is sent, along with live audio, in real-time to your smart device, and parents can share the information with as many caregivers as they like.

Let's start with the possible health concerns of a system like this. Mimo's description of Bluetooth Low Energy as "the safest technology available" is not the same as saying it's categorically safe. Importantly, the phrase "low energy" doesn't refer to the strength of the radio-frequency signal emitted by the device; in fact, BLE chips have the same transmission range as standard Bluetooth chips. Instead, what the term "low energy" refers to is the amount of power the chip consumes. Devices that use Bluetooth Low Energy chips can function much longer on the same size battery, which obviously offers benefits to both manufacturers and consumers. However, it doesn't eliminate the potential concerns of putting another radio-frequency emitting device in close proximity to your infant.

The Mimo system, of course, raises the usual bog standard assortment of privacy concerns: data collection, analysis, anonymization, re-purposing, *etc.* Anytime a product or app offers to produce a colorful graph of data involving your child, it is important to look carefully at how that data is collected, where it is analyzed, and what will be done with it. If you're too bleary-eyed or sleep-deprived to make sense of a company's privacy policy, then you might want to rethink your purchase and use of the product.

There's a little bit of irony in saying this, but one of the great accumulators and analyzers of personal consumer data — Amazon — is also a terrific source of information about various baby products you might be considering. For instance, among Mimo's 60-odd reviews (the product earns 3 out of 5 stars) are concerns about customer service, the ability of the "lilypad" to connect to home WiFi, the use of Bluetooth in infant clothing, the need to make sure your baby is wearing the Mimo onesy whenever it falls asleep, and so on. To be fair, many parents love the product and the information it provides. But no one, as far as I can tell, is particularly worried about the privacy implications.

"Every Breath You Take..."

If products like the Hatch Baby or Mimo don't raise your privacy hackles, then the next generation of infant technology surely will.

Many first-time parents have a healthy dose of insecurity about whether they are doing enough or the right thing for their newborn, especially given the fact the children being born today will need to prosper in an increasingly competitive world. One product that is aimed directly at the sweet spot of nerve-wracked parental worry is the Starling, a device designed to make sure that your baby hears a sufficient number of words during its first few months and years.

As the company's slickly-designed Web site points out, there is a growing body of research that links the amount parents talk to their infant with the speed with which the child develops language skills. The sales pitch takes it from there:

> Even though you don't remember it, your trajectory was set during the earliest years of your life. Studies show that more words heard from birth to age 4 means a child will talk earlier and read sooner. This, in turn, leads to better grades in school, more college scholarship money, and even a better job one day. All from a little small talk!

But here's the catch, according to the company: "Most parents overestimate how much they talk to their children, and since most parent-child interaction happens within a home, it's nearly impossible for families to compare themselves to their peers." Not surprisingly, the company has a solution: a small flower-shaped device that you clip on your child's clothing called the Starling. As you talk to your child, the Starling listens and counts the number of words you say to your infant, the length of time you spending talking, your baby's activity level, and whether it's night or day.

In its privacy policy, the company assures users that it does not record conversations; "It's like listening to a foreign language," the company says. "You can tell that something is being said but you do not know what is being said or who is speaking." Assuming that is true, then the privacy implications of using the Starling itself are minimal. And in the general scheme of things, the amount of personal data the company collects through registration seems pretty limited.

But even if the Starling is not a significant violator of personal privacy right now, parents should always keep in mind how quickly both technology and corporate business plans can change. In its FAQ, Sterling hinted that someday it may move past beyond mere word counting: "We've gone to the edge of speech processing and artificial intelligence and then jumped over it. The thought of 'simply' counting words on a battery-powered wearable device seemed impossible when we first started, but here we are."

There's certainly no technical impediment to recording everything that is said in the vicinity of an Internet-connected microphone; it's merely a function of digital storage space, of which there is a growing abundance worldwide. And more and more consumer devices are being sold with those types of microphones. For my last birthday, for instance, I was given an Amazon Echo, which listens constantly for the word "Alexa." When it hears the word, the device exits low power-mode and prepares to respond to questions or commands like "What's the weather?" or "Set a timer for 30 minutes." Is Amazon listening recording and analyzing every sound in my apartment? I really doubt it, but as I said, the impediments are more practical than technological.

Then there's the talking "Hello Barbie," a $75 version of the classic doll that records what children say to it, uploads the statements to the cloud, and uses those recordings to shape its verbal responses to the child. Needless to say, a lot of parents are justifiably freaked out about this. Anyone who has read Henry Harrison's 50-year-old but chillingly foresighted short story, "I Always Do What Teddy Says," will understand why.

Wholly apart from the profound privacy and child development issues raised by the Mattel product, there are significant security issues as well:

the child-advocacy organization known as the Campaign for Commercial-Free Childhood (CCFC) warned that the collected conversations and related child information could be an attractive targets for hackers. [14.3] Given the endless number of news stories about data hacks, parents should think long and hard about exposing their child to unsupervised interaction with a corporation's profit-driven algorithms.

There's one other aspect of the Starling that may be potentially problematic. The device is built around the idea that at a minimum, newborns should hear 20,000 words per day. In fact, the company has a chart, which I suspect is not closely supported by actual science, that basically predicts certain educational outcomes depending on the number of words parents say to their child:

- Up to 5,000: "More Parent Words"
- 5K - 10K: "Early Talker"
- 10K - 15K: "Early Reader"
- 15K - 20K: "Straight-A Student"
- 20K - 25K: "College Scholarship"
- 25K - 30K: "Unlimited Possibilities"

As my wife pointed out, this basically turns the Starling into the verbal equivalent of a Fitbit. How many parents, she wondered, will try to keep their infant awake at night so that they can hit the 20,000 word mark before the poor kid falls asleep? And what about the quality of the words? Since the Starling apparently is not listening for content, any nonsense syllables will work, but how exactly does that help with college admission? Would it be better to simply leave National Public Radio on all day?

Look, I don't have any disagreement with the idea that it is good for parents to talk and read to their children. There are also a large number of studies that link achievement to the number of books in the house, although those studies probably will have to be re-done for the e-book era. What I think is worrisome is the attempt to quantify and apply external metrics to that type of parent-child interaction. Ideally, parents should be motivated by a desire to interact with their children and not because others in their social network are x thousands of spoken words ahead of them on any given day. But it doesn't take a Ph.D. in sociology to know that is exactly what will happen if the Starling or products like it become popular.

Apps for Tracking and Toys for Educating(?) Your Infant

If you visit most parenting Web sites, it's easy to start wondering exactly how parents ever raised children without the help of Silicon Valley; I'm sure many programmers wonder the same thing as well. Virtually every major parenting resource has articles with some variation of the following headlines:

- "10 Best Baby Apps for New Parents, From Baby Monitors to Lullabies";
- "8 Must-Have Apps For New Parents"
- "10 Essential Apps for New Parents"
- "10 Best Apps for Parents Right Now"

These apps do offer new parents a wide variety of information about infancy and many of them do offer features that can save time, provide reassurance, help preserve memories, track various aspects of a newborn's growth and development, or some combination of all of them. For instance, the app **Baby Connect**, which shows up on a number of these lists, allows parents and caregivers to track a huge range of information about a child, including feedings, nursing, naps, diapers, milestones, pumping, the baby's mood, temperature, what kind of game he's playing, his GPS location, last medicine or vaccine, weight, height, head size, *etc.* It is an exhaustive — and exhausting — list.

Other apps offer more specific features. Some provide different types of monitoring, typically sound or video, through an iPhone. Others, like **babyshusher**, can play calming noises that are supposed to remind the baby of being in the womb. You can even record your own shushing noise for the app to play. You also can find specialized apps for tracking only the data you actually care about, including diaper changes, feeding, growth, and so on. There are also a number of apps that are basically mobile versions of parenting books; both Parenting and WebMD offer good versions of those types of apps.

As a user of a large number of apps myself, I'm certainly not going to try to tell new parents that there is something intrinsically wrong with using a smartphone to assist with parenting. But there are some issues that expecting moms and dads should definitely discuss before deciding to download any particular app.

Will You Actually Use it?

The lead-in to one of the app lists offers this cheery summary for new moms:

> A baby means you need (and deserve!) the best help that mama can get, and sometimes that's an app. Between battling lack of sleep, dirty diapers, nighttime feedings and doctor visits, and all the while trying to record your babe's milestones, if you live off your smart phone or tablet, you'll want to download these apps to help you manage it all. [14.4]

The question, however, is not which app will "help you manage it all." The real question is whether it makes sense to commit to using an app that requires persistent data entry in order to make it effective. Given all of the challenges of parenting, particularly in the first few month's of your child's life, you will quickly learn the difference between "labor-saving" and "labor-creating." Many of the apps in these top 8-10-15 "must-have" lists are in the latter category and not the former.

Have You Read the Privacy Policy?

As I have said repeatedly throughout this book, one of the overarching concerns with respect to any infant-related product is privacy. Manufacturers, retailers, and software publishers will dangle all kinds of advantages and benefits in front of nervous and tech-obsessed parents but all too often, the currency that pays for those benefits is personal information. Before you start loading information about your child into an app, you should take some time to review the publisher's privacy policy and decide if you are comfortable with how your child's information will be stored and used. My personal recommendation is for new parents to start slowly and only share personal information about their child with individuals who are legally required to protect it — chiefly medical professionals and government officials. Beyond that, I think the less capturing and sharing of information the better. There is plenty of time in the years ahead for you and your child to become the target of aggressive marketers.

Will It Distract You from Your Child?

As kids themselves point out, parents in the smartphone era are already too distracted and are not paying enough attention to them. If you are an expecting mom or dad, the odds are good that you also are part of the millennial generation, which means that you already spend a ridiculous amount of time each day using your smartphone or other digital device. As you may already have discovered or soon will, infants also take up a ridiculous amount of time each day. Something has to give, and a lot of people are worried that infants are losing out to Instagram, Facebook, Pokémon Go, or whatever the latest app fad may be. The question to ask yourselves is whether it makes sense to have yet another reason, however virtuous, to interact with your phone instead of your child. Yes, it can be comforting to know that the diapers of your little bundle of joy are squarely in the middle of the bell curve generated by every other use of the app. On the other hand, your weekly or biweekly visits to your pediatrician will do far more to gauge the health of your child and detect any potential problems then the most fastidious data entry in a smartphone app.

Here's an important motto to keep in mind: "Quantity of Data Does Not Mean Quality of Life." Don't get so caught up trying to quantify life that you forget to live it.

Are Hackers Watching Your Baby Sleep?

There is one other question that new and expecting moms need to ask each other: "Do You Actually Know How to Secure the Technology You Use?" For the last several years, a number of tech writers, including yours truly, have been warning that Internet-connected baby monitors are vulnerable to hacking. In 2013, for instance, the Chinese-manufactured Foscam brand was found to have a glaring security hole that allowed hackers to gain access to the audio and video feeds transmitted by the cameras. Forbes technology writer Kashmir Hill estimated that at least 40,000 Foscam monitors were potentially vulnerable. [14.5]

When news of the vulnerability broke, Foscam promptly issued a firmware update, but limited its notification to a relatively unpublicized blog post that said nothing about the potential for hacking. As a result, many if not most Foscam baby monitor owners remain unaware of the risk that strangers might be watching or listening to their children.

Needless to say, it can be deeply upsetting to discover that a stranger might be observing your newborn. In the spring of 2015, a couple in Washington told CBS News that they heard a voice coming out of the monitor saying "Wake up little boy, daddy's looking for you." Their 3-year-old son had been complaining of voices at night, but the couple thought that it was just a function of his imagination. [14.6]

A few weeks earlier, a Rochester, Minnesota family heard music coming out of their child's bedroom. When the parents walked in, the music stopped. The mother looked up the IP address that accessed the device and was able to trace it to Amsterdam before the trail ran cold. [14.7]

And in November 2014, the BBC published a particularly thorough investigation of webcam hacks, including baby monitors. Among other things, the BBC report identified a Russian Web site (since shut down) that gave visitors access to video feeds from over 70,000 unsecured Internet-connected cameras around the world, many of which were located in private homes. [14.8]

These reports should be considered an early warning sign of the potential problems that will plague the roll-out of the much-ballyhooed "Internet of Things." There are powerful forces driving the push to connect more and more physical objects to the Internet, but it will take careful planning and constant vigilance to minimize the risks associated with an IP-infused world. While connected technology can offer some powerful benefits for the parents of newborns, it may be better for your peace of mind to stick with slightly "dumber" parenting tools that reduce the risk of privacy invasions. So far, at least, we have not developed better developmental tools than love, attention, interaction, eye-to-eye contact, and lots of hugs.

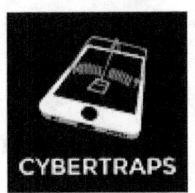

Chapter Fifteen

Parenting in the Era of Digital Devices

After 23 years in Burlington, Vermont, my wife and I moved to Brooklyn, NY, where we rented the second floor of a classic New York brownstone building. On warmer days, like many of our neighbors, we'd often sit on the front stoop in the early evening and watch the world go by.

During the three-plus years we lived there, I noticed a disturbing trend: as young parents push baby carriages and strollers up and down the street, more and more of them were not interacting with their young children but instead were staring at smartphones or tablets. In some cases, the infant was asleep and I can empathize with what I would describe as Periodic Onset Parental Boredom (POPB). But all too often, sadly, the child was staring bright-eyed up at an Apple or Samsung logo rather than their loving parent's face.

This is not a trend that is unique to Brooklyn. I've seen similar scenes in airports, coffee shops, sidewalks, and playgrounds across the United States. But regardless of where it occurs, it is a growing and serious problem that can have long-term effects on our children.

In the previous chapter, I talked about some of the concerns that are associated with so-called "smart" devices like the Hatch Baby or the Starling. One thing that can be said for those products, however, is that their "smartness" doesn't diminish parent/child contact; as unpleasant as the task may be, you still need to change your newborn's diapers, and talking to your kids is almost always a plus, even if a device is busy counting how many words you say. Contrast those devices, however, with another so-called "smart" baby product, the 4moms MamaRoo.

The MamaRoo, which looks roughly like the captain's chair in "Star Trek: The Next Generation" or the floating Barcaloungers in "Wall-E," is an adjustable seat that "can rock your baby in various patterns at a few different speed levels," play various soothing sounds, and entertain your baby with an mobile suspended over his or her head. The chair connects via Bluetooth to a smartphone app that allows you to "control the volume, select the sound effects, adjust the movement speed, and choose the movement pattern that the chair uses to rock your child." [15.1]

Let's be clear: I am not suggesting that parents should never put their infant in a baby seat, bouncy chair, or even swing, although it is worth noting that the American Association of Pediatrics does strongly discourage parents from letting infants or babies sleep in an upright or semi-upright position. [15.2] It's not possible to hold your infant 24/7, and every parent needs occasional hands-free moments during the course of the day. But any time you add electronics to the mix, as the MamaRoo does, then the potential exists that the electronics will distract a parent from necessary childcare or diminish parent-child interaction.

That's not a tremendous risk with MamaRoo, to be fair. The app and baby chair have a limited number of motion and sound settings, so the potential for adult digital distraction is low. But as this chapter demonstrates, there are many compelling reasons to reduce electronic distractions as much as possible when infants or young children are nearby and under your supervision.

The Risks of Distracted Parenting

As I mentioned earlier, while I was researching and writing this book over the summer of 2016, the game Pokémon Go was released and become a overnight global phenomenon. One man named Nick Johnson walked all over New York City for hours at a time (often until 4 or 5 in the morning) to become the first person to capture all of the Pokémon available in the United States. When his feat was reported in the news, Marriott Rewards and Expedia offered to sponsor Johnson on trips to Paris, Hong Kong, and Sydney so that he could catch three rare Pokémon characters that only "live" in those parts of the world. [15.3]

While perhaps a tad obsessive, Johnson's quest presumably had little impact on the people around him, apart from his apparently supportive girlfriend, who hopefully got to accompany him on at least one of his overseas Pokémon excursions. But what if in your zeal to hunt down the elusive Wartotle, Clefairy, or Wigglytuff, you overlook the fact that you have a real, live child?

That's apparently what happened to Brent and Brianne Daley, an Arizona couple that left their 2-year-old son sleeping in their San Tan Valley home while they went out looking for Pokémon Go characters. Unfortunately, the little boy woke up while they were gone and was discovered wandering around outside at 10:30pm in 95 degree weather. When neighbors saw that he was stuck outside and couldn't get back in his house, they called the police. Officers helped the boy get into the unlocked house, waited there for the parents to return, and then promptly arrested them on charges of child endangerment. [15.4]

The Daleys, you no doubt are thinking to yourself, are an extreme case. There's no way, you reassure yourself, that I would leave a small child at home alone while I wander around the neighborhood looking for imaginary creatures on my smartphone. And in all likelihood, that's true. But think about how many times during the day you glance away from what you are doing to look at your smartphone so that you can answer a text, send an email, update Facebook, post a photo of your child to Instagram and read the responses, search Yelp for someplace to eat dinner, or any of a hundred other short but still-distracting tasks? Those types of micro-distractions don't grab the headlines in quite the same way as the Daleys did, but under the wrong set of circumstances, the consequences can be even more severe.

Physical Injury

If you are so utterly immersed in playing Pokémon Go on your smartphone that you trip on a curb and break your wrist trying to catch yourself, it's unfortunate. No doubt you will feel pain and probably some embarrassment, either because people see it happen or you later are compelled to explain the epically stupid cause of your injury. But if you manage to overlook the fact that you have a child, or you get into an accident while your child is in your car or a stroller, then the consequences of smartphone distraction escalate quickly from the merely unfortunate to the truly tragic.

As we saw in Chapter Two, people who try to use their phones while walking or driving run a significantly elevated risks of badly injuring or even killing someone, or even themselves, in an accident. Pretty much everything is more complicated and requires more attention when a child is present. It is difficult to overstate just how much physical attention and supervision children need, from the moment they are born until they finally are old enough to appreciate and safely navigate the world's physical risks on their own. In the summer of 2016, the Child Accident Prevention Trust (CAPT) in the United Kingdom made "Turn off technology for safety" for the theme of the organization's Child Safety Week.

> No-one can watch over their little ones 100% of the time, but not being distracted by technology at crucial times of the day and in certain hectic situations is one of the simple measures

parents and carers can reduce the risk for children and pressure on themselves.

Switching your phone off or to silent say from 5-6pm, is not a big ask, but it means one less distraction for busy parents. It also gives children the message that they are the focus. And it sets a good example to children and young people that it is good to turn off at times when you need to concentrate to stay safe, like crossing the road.

CAPT was motivated to focus on distraction by a study it conducted that showed that nearly twenty-five percent of parents were unaware that their child was in or nearly in an accident because the parent was focusing on his or her phone instead. Dr. Rahul Chodhari, a senior pediatrician at the Royal College of Paediatrics and Child Health, spearheaded the investigation and underscored just how quickly things could go wrong:

Accidents often happen when we're distracted and mobile phones are increasingly to blame — whether it's a teenager stepping out into traffic while instant messaging or a baby grabbing at a hot drink or biting into a liquitab while their parent is replying to a text.

It only takes a split second for an accident to happen so I urge parents and young people to adapt their behaviour. [15.5]

Digital devices are not the only source of distraction for parents, of course. A study of randomly-selected children and their caregivers in New York City playgrounds found that the most common distraction in that environment was talking to other adults (33%), with electronic devices being a close second (30%). Just under one-third of the children engaged in what the researchers defined as "risky" behavior, ranging from walking up a slide to jumping off moving swings. Not surprisingly, "[c]hildren whose caregivers were distracted were significantly more likely to engage in risky behaviors." [15.6]

Just as with pedestrian injuries, there is data showing that the number of child injuries is climbing in parallel to increases in cellphone usage. According to the parenting blog Kars4Kids, the number of nonfatal injuries to children rose by 12% between 2007 and 2010; injuries on playground equipment increased by 17%, while accidents involving nursery room equipment climbed a disturbing 31%. During that same period of time, smartphone use rose from 6% to 30%. [15.7] It's not difficult to draw the logical conclusion.

The "Brexting" Controversy

One of the things you will quickly realize, if you haven't already, is that the Internet is not a judgment-free zone; in fact, quite the opposite. We would certainly all be better off if we observed some variation of the rule, "Troll not, lest ye be trolled." But notwithstanding the basic principles that should guide all our interactions, both online and off, you will undoubtedly find any number of people willing and eager to judge the parenting skills and choices you demonstrate in any photo you post online. Perhaps that might make you think twice about posting photos or videos online, but that's obviously a decision you and your partner will need to make for yourselves.

One topic that is absolutely guaranteed to get Mrs. Grundy up in arms is breastfeeding. There are few parenting topics that are more hotly debated and about which people have such deep-seated opinions. Breast or bottle? Breastfeed in public or only in private? The list goes on. And now social media has added new layers to the controversies. Should breastfeeding photos be censored? Many social media platforms have wrestled with this, including Facebook and Instagram. Should mothers even post them in the first place?

Here's a good example of just how judgmental the Web can get. Over the past year, thanks largely to social media, a new controversy has arisen. Women who post photos of themselves using a smartphone while breastfeeding their child are now being publicly shamed for engaging in a practice dubbed "brexting." The strained portmanteau was coined sometime earlier in the year, but it really began to attract media attention following an appearance by psychologist Katayune Kaeni on Southern California Public Radio in September 2015.

Dr. Kaeni, who specializes in maternal mental health, drew a bright line in the sand regarding the use of smartphones while breastfeeding.

> When babies are first born their vision is only basically from the breast to the mother's face. That's as far as they can see. So babies do a lot of staring and bonding in that way. [If a mother is on her smartphone, she] could be missing cues that they're full or they're still hungry or their latch isn't secure or if they are having trouble swallowing. [15.8]

The debate falls along predictable lines. Many mothers agree with Dr.

Kaeni that breastfeeding is a uniquely intimate opportunity for mother and newborn to bond, and that any use of a device, watching television or even reading a book interferes with the bonding process. Other mothers strongly reject the public shaming and argue that a little texting or Instagram while a baby is feeding and drifting off to sleep at 3 in the morning is not exactly child abuse. My favorite quote on the subject came from a mother writing for CafeMom's blog, The Stir: "If the phone can help a mom stay up during those oh-so-wonderful late-night feedings, who am I to judge? My husband isn't going to wake up and entertain me." [15.9]

Rebecca Naylor, the CEO of the Australian Breastfeeding Association, offers a particularly rational perspective on this debate. It's one that applies to many parenting-technology debates:

> It's in fact all about balance. Sometimes breastfeeding will be a more intense process, and sometimes it will be less so. Women are people and so inevitably they are not going to spent every single moment of feeding their child staring lovingly at them. Sometimes they'll be distracted by their phones, by other toddlers or the TV; at other times they will be more focused. While it is true that breastfeeding is about more than just the nutrition — it is an emotional connection between mother and child - we have to be careful about putting too much pressure on mothers to be perfect. One way one mother feeds their child will be different to how another feeds theirs. [15.10]

The Eyes Have It

It is certainly quite common for new parents to wonder about whether they have the skills to properly raise a happy and successful child. It is a completely normal worry and one that thankfully fades quickly as you get more experienced in caring for your child. By the time the second or third rolls around, you'll find yourself freely handing out advice, as this book demonstrates. But there is no question that the early days of parenthood are a bit daunting. Fortunately, it turns out that one of the best steps you can take to promote your child's long-term emotional and intellectual well-being is also one of the least complicated: simply pay attention.

I definitely agree that there is too much finger-pointing and shaming online. That being said, the digital scolds are not completely wrong. Expecting moms and dads should take some time to think about their technology use and the impact that it might be having on the development of their new child. From the earliest moments of its life, Dr. Kaeni warns, your child's competition with your device for attention may be shaping his or her behavior.

> If baby is trying to make contact with you by noises or smiles and they can't and they learn over time that they can't rely on you to respond, it runs the risk of them becoming either anxiously attached to your or insecurely attached to you and they will ramp up their behavior until you pay attention. [15.11]

Behavioral issues are not the only possible by-product of distracted parenting and lack of eye contact — your smartphone may also damage your child's future academic ability. According to researchers at the Indiana University Department of Psychological and Brain Sciences, if caregivers are distracted while playing with children, there is a good chance that they will raise children with shorter attention spans themselves.

The researchers equipped toddlers and caregivers with head-mounted cameras that could track the line of vision and eye movements of both, and then asked them to play together using a variety of physical toys. They concluded that when the caregivers focused on a particular toy for more than 3.6 seconds, then the child would focus on the same object for 2.3 seconds longer, even after the caregiver stopped looking at it. Ultimately, the researchers concluded that focused caregivers helped children concentrate on a particular toy or object up to four times longer.

The lead researcher, Professor Chen Yu, said that even a few seconds of additional focus per play session can add up to significant benefits over a period of months and years:

> The ability of children to sustain attention is known as a strong indicator for later success in areas such as language acquisition, problem-solving and other key cognitive development milestones. Caregivers who seem distracted or whose eyes wander a lot while their children play appear to negatively impact infants' burgeoning attention spans during a key stage of development.

The study classified attention span development in response to three different types of child-caregiver interactions: The best development occurred when adults allowed the child to lead the play, and then focused on the object with the child; a lower level of development — but still positive — occurred when adults tried to lead the play by encouraging the infants to play with toys the adults selected; and the least development resulted when adults failed to interact with the infants at all or were quickly distracted by their phones or something else in the room.

As Professor Yu put it somewhat dryly, "When you've got someone who isn't responsive to a child's behavior, it could be a real red flag for future problems." [15.12]

The take-away from this, obviously, is that adult attempts at multitasking may actively impede your child's own ability to develop a reasonable attention span. Obviously, an occasional interruption is not going to ruin your child's future academic success but if your phone or other digital device gets more of your eye contact then your infant, then it may worth considering whether there is some way to restructure the time you spend with your newborn.

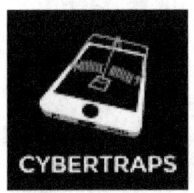

Chapter Sixteen
Delaying Your Child's First Use of Technology

In theory, there should be a significant gap between the parenting concerns discussed in *Cybertraps for Expecting Moms and Dads* and the issues I discussed in *Cybertraps for the Young*, which covers the legal risks that older kids face from the use and misuse of digital devices. But that gap is shrinking rapidly; according to recent surveys, the average age at which a child first uses an electronic device is now below 1 year, and manufacturers seem determined to push that age even lower.

One of the standard slides that I use in my lectures for educators and parents shows a variety of products designed to expose infants to digital technology, including mobiles that can hold a smartphone and bouncy chairs equipped with a tablet stand. While that slide always gets a good laugh from attendees — they particularly like the picture of the potty training chair with the built-in tablet computer — it also elicits some gasps of dismay. While there is no serious disagreement that that today's children need to know how to use technology, many are shocked to see such a concerted effort by retailers to put digital devices in front of such tiny faces.

Unfortunately, as with so many of the other issues I've discussed in this book, the use of technology by infants and toddlers is fiercely debated and generally raises more questions than answers. Part of the problem is that in many ways, we are still in the early stages of understanding both the physiology and psychology of human development. Even as we struggle to better understanding the basic factors that contribute to a happy and successful childhood, we are introducing a host of new devices and content delivery tools that influence development in ways that we have just begun to study and assess. To one degree or another, every childhood is a long-running experiment, but as with so much else, technology has the capacity to accelerate both benefits and potential harms.

Can the Future Be Baby-Proofed?

Given how much we use our phones and other digital devices while we try to do other things, like feeding an infant, the most immediate concern for expecting moms and dads is to avoid injuring your newborn with your favorite device. This may seem like an obvious issue, but it is not a trivial concern. By their very nature, mobile devices tend not to stay in one place, safely out of the reach of little hands. Part of the requisite baby-proofing of your home involves thinking about where devices will be kept, how you will use them near your child, and how much access your child will have to them. A horrified post by a new mother to an online baby community helps to illustrate one of the risks:

> I dropped my iPhone on my baby!!!!!!
>
> I'm so upset. LO was sleeping on my chest and he looked soooo sweet and I wanted to capture the moment, so I took my phone and lifted it way over my head to get a picture of the two of us and I dropped it and it fell right onto my baby's head! And you know those things aren't light, especially falling like 18 inches or more!
>
> He started screaming! He only cried for like a minute then he cuddled up with his paci. When DH came home I was crying hysterically, scared that I gave him a concussion or something. But DH said that he's fine. There's no bump or bruise or anything. But still, I can't believe I did that. I'm so sad.
>
> I love LO sooooo much, I'm just crazy about him, and seeing him hurt kills me and I can't believe I'm the one who hurt him. I feel awful and I'm scared that I really damaged him! [16.1]

LO no doubt is grateful that his mother was not trying to take his photo with an iPad. Fortunately, his mother was able to report to other members of the online community, many of whom shared similar incidents, that he suffered no ill effects. Still, it's not something that most pediatricians would recommend.

In a surprisingly short period of time, your child will transition from being an almost totally immobile newborn to an increasingly mobile toddler. As they start to pull themselves up and trundle around your house, you will find that they regularly grab at objects and pull them off tables, couches, and chairs. They chew on random objects, particularly when teething. As they get a little older, they like to drop, throw, whack, and kick things. All of these typical behaviors carry some risk of injury, depending on what is in your house, but the metal cases, glass screens, and occasional sharp edges of digital devices can be particularly painful if they drop from a height onto your unsuspecting child.

Your primary concern, obviously, should be the safety and physical well-being of your child. But as more and more electronic devices are put in front of toddlers or in their grubby little hands, it's worth remembering that the devices themselves are not invincible.

The reality is that newborns and little kids are inherently messy; they spit up and spill things with regularity and sometimes with enthusiasm. Neither body fluids nor mashed peas, or whatever the purée of the day may be, are helpful to high-end electronics. At the very least, you might want to think about whether you can easily replace your iPad or Samsung tablet and its data in the event your little bundle of joy decides to regurgitate the morning feeding all over it.

Possible Physical Risks of Infant Use of Technology

Accidents by their very nature are unpredictable. While you certainly don't want to drop your phone on your newborn, you can take steps to minimize the chances of that happening. More importantly, you know that bouncing your iPhone of his forehead is not part of the normal operation of the device. What should be of greater concern is whether the innate operation of these devices — *i.e.*, using them exactly as they are designed — may someday result in physical or developmental problems for your child. Again, because our use of mobile technology is so recent (the iPhone is just about to turn 10), there are no firm answers. But there are a number of issues you should discuss with your pediatrician.

Does Radiation Pose a Greater Risk to Infants?

Throughout this book, I've talked about the potential impact of having radiation-emitting devices near sensitive parts of our bodies. Let me reiterate that there is considerable debate about whether any of our digital devices, particularly smartphones, are in fact causing any damage at all. After talking to your physician, you can decide for yourself what level of risk is acceptable to you personally. But while you can have a conversation with your doctor, your newborn child cannot, so you'll need to do that for her.

Four years ago, the American Academy of Pediatrics (AAP) asked the Federal Communications Commission (FCC) to reconsider its standards for radiation absorption from cell phones in light of the fact that more and more young children are using those devices. [16.2] As the AAP's then-president Dr. Robert Block pointed out, the FCC standards were designed to calculate safe exposure limits for adults, not children. In a letter to the FCC, Dr. Block argued that children are much more vulnerable:

> Children, however, are not little adults and are disproportionately impacted by all environmental exposures, including cell phone radiation. In fact, according to [the International Agency for Research on Cancer], when used by children, the average RF energy deposition is two times higher in the brain and 10 times higher in the bone marrow of the skull, compared with mobile phone use by adults.

To date, however, the FCC has not made any adjustments to its recommended specific absorption rates for cell phones.

Most newborns and infants are not cell phone users, so this is not an immediate area of concern for parents. However, you may want to think about where you hold your phone if you decide to engage in a little 'brexting.' Of more immediate concern to some parents are the possible effects of transmission technologies that are more likely to be in regular proximity to your newborn: WiFi and Bluetooth.

Once again, the debate in this area has gotten fairly heated (pun intended). In January 2015, *Forbes* summarized a "controversial" study entitled "Why children absorb more microwave radiation than adults: The consequences." [16.3] The study, which consisted of a survey of prior literature, was published in the *Journal of Microscopy and Ultrastructure*, and concluded in part that "[t]he risk to children and adolescent from exposure to microwave radiating devices is considerable. Adults have a smaller but very real risk, as well." [16.4] Concerns like these recently led France to ban the use of WiFi in nurseries, despite virtually no serious evidence of a link between WiFi and harm to humans. [16.5]

For additional information from the anti-radiation side of the debate, you can view a collection of other exposure studies, along with disturbing lists of potential health effects, on a number of different Web sites. One particularly emphatic site, run by a British organization, is called Wired Child. The group describes itself as follows:

> WiredChild is a charity run by a group of concerned parents, raising awareness of the potential risks to children of exposure to radiation from mobile phones and other wireless technology. We hope to enable other parents, schools and children achieve a better balance between safety and convenience.

We want to increase awareness of the extent of the evidence of serious risk, and the simple ways to reduce those risks. We hope to head off a potential increase in cancers and other serious illnesses amongst the generation of children growing up today.

These types of concerns, however, are flatly rejected by most scientists. Some question the quality of the anti-radiation research; the study cited by Forbes, for instance, was criticized for its lack of original research and less-than-credible source. [16.6] Others point to basic principles of science in dismissing concerns. As I discussed in Chapter One, the frequencies and intensity of both WiFi and Bluetooth are well below any levels found to be harmful so far. One of the better summations of these basic principles occurred on the entertaining and informative Web site, How-To Geek. In response to the question "Could Wi-Fi Be Harmful to a Newborn Baby?," one reader replied in part:

Perfectly safe.

The term "radiation" is often used to scare people. Let's get it straight. There are two factors – frequency and intensity. Frequency has a far larger effect on how damaging radiation is. Wi-Fi and other radio communications use a very low frequency – far below visible light.

…

Apart from frequency, there is intensity. Non-ionizing radiation can also be damaging – but this really only applies to higher intensities. And ionizing radiation is not always dangerous – our bodies can cope with lower intensities, which is why we don't all die in the sun (vampires are another matter). Wi-Fi has a transmitting power usually far under 1 Watt (I've seen figures for 200 mW). And most of that energy never reaches you – by the inverse square law, you only get about 1/distance squared of that. In layman's terms – the energy spreads equally in all directions. 10 meters away? 1/100 * 200 mW = 2 mW. That's *nothing*. [16.7]

If you come away from your research and your conversation with your pediatrician that these types of non-ionizing radiation pose a virtually non-existent threat to your child — which is the position taken by the vast majority of scientists who have studied the issue — then have fun equipping your child with the latest and greatest digital devices. But even if the risk is negligible, there certainly is no harm in thinking twice or even a third time about whether the alleged benefits make the expense and exposure worthwhile.

The Impact of Technology on Infant Vision

The odds are good that within the first year of your child's life, he or she will begin using a digital device. It might be the latest educational toy, or a new app that promises rapid language acquisition, or simply a tablet with a streaming video so that you can actually make dinner. While those may all seem like good justifications, there are a couple of different risks that should be considered first.

A couple of years ago, Dr. Jim Kokkinakis, a Sydney-based optometrist, reported that his practice had seen steep increases in the number of patients with eye strain and dry eyes resulting from too much time staring at a screen. He warned that children face an additional risk: damage to the retina resulting from excessive exposure to the intense blue light emitted by light emitting diode (LED) screens. [16.8]

The problem, Dr. Kokkinakis said, is that the eyes of children allow much more blue light to reach the retina compared to adults. Over time, that exposure might result in macular degeneration and an earlier onset of cataracts. Dr. Kokkinakis said he now routinely adds a blue light blocking filter to prescription lenses for children and recommends that all children wear "screen lenses" (the indoor equivalent of sunglasses) when using a computer or mobile screen.

> What worries me is we are giving tablets and phones to children as young as two to play with and over years we really don't know what the ramifications might be. Unfortunately we are going to be experts in hindsight.

The concerns of Dr. Kokkinakis were echoed last fall in a paper published by a team of Irish researchers in *Psychology Research*. Among other things, the scientists underscored the ongoing need for further research into the effects of blue light "on the undeveloped eye sight of infants and toddlers."

> The blue light from smartphones and tablets is known to cause long term damage, although the extent of the damage is still unknown. If blue light can negatively impact fully developed eyes, it is important to investigate what impact this light is

having on the undeveloped eye sight of infants and toddlers. [16.9]

It is not just the quality of light that is issue. A related concern is how close an infant or toddler's eyes are to the screen. For nearly fifteen years, optometrists have warned that school-aged kids are reporting a variety of vision-related problems, including headaches, eye soreness, and blurry vision. All of those symptoms can contribute to nearsightedness, also known as myopia. [16.10] Of course, a condition like myopia can have multiple causes, so it would be unfair to blame technology alone. Nonetheless, there appears to be a growing amount of evidence showing a linkage between the amount of a child's screen time and his or her vision health. As the Irish doctors noted, this is also a particular concern for our youngest children:

> Until they develop fully, an infant's visual acuity is limited. Spending a lot of time looking at screens close-up can cause myopia (short or near-sightedness) and this can occur because children are not spending sufficient time looking at things that are in the distance.

In my lectures to parents and educators, I urge adults to delay child use of electronics as long as possible, in part because of the issues raised by these researchers and in part because those same children will inevitably spend large amounts of time looking at device screens in the years to come, whether at home, in school, at work or, most likely, all three. Our eyeballs did not evolve to spend hours every day staring at a light-emitting object a foot or less from our face, so delaying the onslaught of electrons can only help.

Developmental Concerns

Possible damage to vision is the most immediate risk for infants and toddlers when they use digital technology. But researchers are worry that devices and apps can alter child development in negative ways. And the percentage of kids in diapers who are using digital technology is skyrocketing. In 2011, according to Common Sense Media, the percentage of kids under 2 who were using mobile devices was just 10% in 2011. Three years later, the percentage had risen to nearly 40%. [16.11] And just last year, a survey conducted in a Philadelphia pediatric clinic found that by the age of 4, **96.4** percent used a mobile device daily. Most had started doing so before the age of 1. Parents reported that the main reasons for giving such young children mobile devices were: 1) to get chores done; 2) to calm the child; and 3) at bedtime, which ironically may have had the opposite effect. [16.12]

Dr. Richard House, a British psychologist and Senior Lecturer in Early Childhood, Department of Education Studies & Liberal Arts, University of Winchester, has gone so far as to say that parents who provide tablets and other digital devices to very young children are committing child abuse. [16.13]

In a world in which some children suffer unconscionable physical and emotional abuse, it's a little difficult to take a statement like that completely seriously. Nonetheless, it is worth thinking about the potential long-term consequences of allowing children to use digital devices at younger and younger ages and for longer and longer periods of time. There are three that I think are particularly consequential.

2D or Not 2D? That Is the Question

The first concern is about the impact that technology might be having on the development of motor skills by our children. Are we destroying the ability of our children to do manual tasks by allowing them to play with technology, or do digital devices and apps actually enhance those skills? Just how important are motor skills anyway?

As with every aspect of child development, the debate over the impact of technology on this aspect of child development is intense. But while we may not know the specific outcome of the debate just yet, there are two relevant facts that seem incontrovertible: First, young children are using digital devices, particularly those with touchscreens, in astounding numbers, and second, the sales of "traditional" analog toys have been falling steadily over the same time period. [16.14]

A child's development of motor skills is one of the key milestones in infancy, because it is directly linked to the child's growing cognitive capabilities. Last summer, Dr. Priscilla Caçola, an assistant professor of kinesiology in the UT Arlington College of Nursing and Health Innovation, helped develop a questionnaire to assist parents in evaluating the types of play spaces and toys most likely to assist a child in the development of gross and fine motor skills. It is worth noting that none of the examples of beneficial toys supplied by the researchers were equipped with screens, touch or otherwise. Professor Caçola underscored the importance of her research:

Developing a child's motor skills is extremely important

because motor development is actually the mediator of cognitive, social and emotional development. Good motor skills predict a whole lot later in life, so it might be something that all of us should be concerned about early in a child's life.

As entertaining as a tablet may be for a 6-month old, the device can do very little to assist in the child's development of motor skills. While educational apps may offer the appearance of manipulation, it's a poor substitute for the real thing. Even as 3-D technology improves dramatically, the interface is intrinsically a 2-D experience, a flat screen with a never-changing texture. Compare that to the wide range of tactile feedback a child gets when playing with blocks, balls, different fabrics, *etc.* All of that data is critically important to the cognitive development of children.

One toy manufacturer that takes a particularly strong stand on this issue is Spielgaben, which produces a sequential series of age-appropriate wooden and fabric toys. The company acknowledges that we and our children live in a digital world, but not surprisingly, offers a number of arguments in support of physical toys. The first, and in many ways the most compelling, is the open-ended possibilities of "real" toys:

> With real physical toys, a child is limited only by their own imaginations and creativity. In an electronic game, a child can only play what has been created for them by programmers. Creativity is stifled through the constant use of digital educational toys. They can only respond to a pre-produced set of experiences with limited options.
>
> A child's choices are limited when it comes to electronic play. When playing with traditional toys, a child can play alone, with a friend, or with an adult. They can use the toy for purposes other than what the original intent was. They can play with the toy in one way, and then change mid-course to do something else with it. None of these scenarios are options when it comes to play with electronic educational games. [16.15]

The Impact on Imagination

It's not surprising that Spielgaben focuses on the importance of imagination. Educators and researchers have been studying the role of play and imagination in the development in children for some time now. There is increasing consensus that free-structured play is not only an important aspect of early childhood but also a valuable attribute throughout school and into adulthood. In 2000, for instance, Dr. Paul Harris, a professor at the Graduate School of Education at Harvard University, published a book entitled *The Work of Imagination*. "Human beings," he told the *Harvard Gazette* a short time later, "have a gift for fantasy, which shows itself at a very early age and then continues to make all sorts of contributions to our intellectual and emotional life throughout the lifespan." [16.16]

Imaginative play offers a number of significant cognitive benefits for developing children: the ability to conceive of different perspectives and recognize differences of opinion; the integration of competing concepts; divergent thinking; the ability to express both positive and negative emotions; the ability to integrate intellectual concepts with emotions; the development of self-regulation; and perhaps most importantly, the development of creativity. [16.17]

Technology can interfere with a child's imagination in ways that are not necessarily immediately obvious. At some point during the last couple of decades, for instance, I heard a radio interview of an older African-American actor, who told a powerful story about the impact of technology on imagination during his childhood. When he was a kid, he said, he would listen to the Lone Ranger on the radio and imagine himself as the hero of the story. But that got harder, he continued, once television was introduced and the networks began telling the same stories on screen. Invariably, the hero — the Lone Ranger, Superman, Batman, whoever — was a white actor. Even in his imagination, the actor said, it was harder and harder to cast himself in the leading role. I am sorry that I can't remember the actor who told that evocative and moving story; both memory and Google have failed me. But his lesson on the power of imagination and the inherently limiting impact of technology has remained with me.

The fundamental issue, as Spielgaben points out, is whether a toy is open-ended or inherently finite. Even if a child is playing a so-called "open-ended" electronic game, such as Minecraft, the overall structure and operation of the game has been determined by the choices made by the programmers. Moreover, every electronic game like Minecraft is played on a device which has a static and two-dimensional interface that offers little or no tactile variation. And of course, from a health perspective, there is a big difference between a child sitting in front of a digital device for hours and spending those same hours engaged in active play. Spend even a small amount of time on medical or parenting Web sites and you'll quickly see that there is serious concern about the rise in childhood obesity due to inactivity.

Given the role that imagination and creativity must play in helping us to solve the deeply challenging problems we face, it is fair to say that we all have a vested interest in encouraging the development of imagination in our children. "[I]t is only through imagination," Bertrand Russell said, "that men become aware of what the world might be; without it, 'progress' would become mechanical and trivial." [16.18] This was neatly echoed two decades later by the playwright George Bernard Shaw in *Back to Methuselah* (and then by Senator Robert Kennedy in 1968): "You see things; and you say 'Why?' But I dream things that never were; and I say 'Why not?'" [16.19]

Can Society Survive without Empathy?

There is one other vitally important role that imagination plays during childhood: it helps to encourage the development of empathy, "the feeling that you understand and share another person's experiences and emotions : the ability to share someone else's feelings. [16.20]

In Chapter Two, I discussed the role that technology is playing in the rise of narcissism among millennials and Gen Z. It's a significant concern, one that can lead to risky behaviors resulting in injury or even death, particularly among older teens and young adults. But there is a parallel phenomenon arising out of early childhood technology use that in the long run, may be much more destructive: a clear and growing deficit of empathy and compassion.

There is some evidence that empathy is an innate quality among many species, including humans; even young infants have been shown to demonstrate empathetic behavior. But researchers also have found that empathy ultimately is the result of socialization by family, friends and community. It is a process that does not fully complete until late adolescence, when our pre-frontal cortex — the portion of our brain in which we assess the impact of our actions on others — slowly comes online.

Empathy is a valuable quality for children to develop, both for their own sake and for the sake of people around them. Children with strong empathy skills, for instance, typically do better in school and in social situations, which can position them for success as they mature into adulthood. Some have gone so far, in fact, as to label empathy as a child's most important skill in the 21st century.

> We are moving away from self-centered and culturally-centric views of the world to embrace our global partners as open, receptive, willing, engaged, empowered counterparts who are ready to move forward together. Efforts to communicate, collaborate, create, innovate, problem-solve and transform will not be successful without global empathy. [16.21]

Parents are the first and most important teachers of empathy to children. The educational process starts from the very earliest moments of life, when parents react to a newborn's cries by comforting, changing, or feeding her. As children age, they learn empathetic behavior by watching their peers and the adults around them. Parents can actively encourage acquisition of empathy by talking about feelings, reading stories that illustrate how others feel, encouraging imagination, and validating the child's own feelings, even when they seem excessive or irrational. [16.22]

Ironically, technology both enhances the need for empathy and makes its acquisition more challenging. Many of the problems that occur online — cyberbullying, trolling, doxxing, electronic sexual assault — are as much about a lack of empathy for the feelings of others as they are about active hostility towards a specific person. One of the main reasons for this is that in most online communications, it is not possible for people to see each other's facial expressions or other physical reactions. As a result, it is much easier for people to say or even do things that they would never do face-to-face.

The lack of empathy online is disturbing enough in its own right. But the real concern is that our increasingly tech-addicted children might not develop empathy at all, or merely some sadly diminished version. The earlier that kids start using devices and the longer they use them, the less time they have to interact with other people in person and the less opportunity they have to develop the skills needed to actually empathize with others. If the child's use of technology is compounded by the fact that parents themselves are absorbed in their devices and are interacting less with their child, then it will be that much harder for the child to acquire this critical skill of connecting on a human level with peers and colleagues.

As this book amply demonstrates, digital technology does not make parenting easier. It raises a host of new issues for parents to debate and discuss. The use of technology by children born today and tomorrow is simply inevitable; digital technology and electronic communications are being woven into every aspect of our lives. The best gift parents can give their children, paradoxically, is to delay their exposure to digital devices for as long as possible. We are slowly learning that a child's earliest, most formative years are an irreplaceable opportunity to develop skills that are much more difficult to acquire later, if at all.

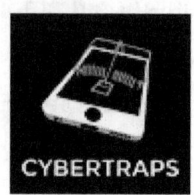

Conclusion

To paraphrase one of my all-time favorite movies, "Bull Durham," parenting, particularly during the first year, is a simple game: You feed the baby, you clean the baby, you hold the baby, you love the baby. Pretty much everything else is just background noise.

But as I hope this book has illustrated, lurking beneath the surface of virtually every technology-related childcare issue are important and legitimate concerns that every new parent should thoughtfully consider. Ideally, those conversations should occur as early as possible during your pregnancy, before the combined forces of aggressive pregnancy marketing, nervousness, and lack of sleep overwhelm you and make you question your judgment.

When you are considering any technology-related decision before, during, and immediately after your pregnancy, there are four main themes to consider: health, safety, privacy, and identity.

Health

While safety issues of course are the real headline grabbers, the most pressing issues regarding digital devices involve your reproductive health and the long-term health of your child. The challenge, unfortunately, is that there are a lot of questions right now and not very many solid answers. We don't know for certain, for instance, what impact digital devices have on our fertility, which in turn may or may not have an impact on our ability to conceive a child in the first place.

The potential health risks to a fetus during pregnancy are just as worrisome. Although the human body has had many millennia of experience in birthing children, we are exposing ourselves to unprecedented biological and technological conditions — and that's even assuming, of course, that millennials are interested in having children or, even more remarkably, are interested in engaging in the intercourse that might conceivably lead to pregnancy. There is little likelihood, of course, that millennials or Generation Z will give up sex or parenthood altogether. However, the trends are not encouraging and the explosion of digital technology over the last three decades — devices, the Web, and apps —

has definitely played a role in distracting younger people.

Needless to say, the health concerns raised by technology do not disappear the moment a child is born; far from it. All of the concerns regarding noise, heat, and radiation apply as much to newborns as to fetuses, if not more so. More importantly, new parents will find themselves under relentless pressure from manufacturers, retailers, and even family and friends to use more and more data-collecting and Internet-connected technology in their parenting, and to provide even very young children with high-tech devices and toys. That pressure should be resisted for as long as is humanly possible.

Even though my years of hands-on parenting are behind me, I fully sympathize with the desire to use whatever tools might be available to ease the relentless and physically draining demands of a newborn infant. Those little bundles of humanity are adorable and lovely and inspiring and utterly precious. They are also demanding and innately self-centered and utterly exhausting. If you have "friends" on social media who tell you otherwise, block them now. It is so, so tempting to invest in anything — Bluetooth-equipped baby seat, body sensor onesies, whatever — that offers the promise of slightly greater peace of mind and the possibility of a few more moments of sleep.

As much as possible, however, those sleep-deprived impulses should be rejected. I really don't think that we are on the cusp or even on the slippery slope of some Huxley-esque dystopia in which each new generation emerges fully-formed and class-assigned from some high-tech birthing pod (fortunately, the name "iPod" has already been used). But there is growing evidence of the negative effects, both physical and emotional, of too much screen time and not enough human face time. One of the single best things that parents can do to help themselves and their children avoid early cybertraps is to limit the amount of time everyone spends looking at screens.

That is particularly true for infants and very young children. Not only do our youngest children benefit the most from eye-to-eye contact with the people around them, but their still-developing eyes are the most sensitive to the bright light generated by tablets and smartphones. Give them a break and wait as long as possible before yielding to their pleas to use the device they see you holding so much.

Safety

The most fundamental question that parents should ask themselves throughout pregnancy and infancy is whether the use of a digital device in any way threatens the safety of a growing fetus or the well-being of a newborn. If you spend some time reviewing parenting Web sites and blogs, as I have over the past year or so, you'll see that there is growing concern about the possibility of misuse of social media photographs. It is true that if you post photos of your adorable child taken with your smartphone and forget to turn off the location data, an individual theoretically could use that information to locate and threaten your family. The chances of that happening, however, are incredibly small.

When we focus our attention on stranger-danger, we often lose sight of the threats posed by our own behaviors. The most clear-cut examples of safety risks for your child involve the use of digital device while driving pregnant, or with your infant in the car. As we've seen, it is only slightly less dangerous to use your digital device while walking or pushing a baby carriage. AT&T's ad campaign is correct: "It can wait."

Similarly, it is important to realize just how quickly your child can get injured or hurt, even in an effectively child-proofed home. You may think that you are only spending a few seconds flipping through Facebook or Instagram, or swiping left and right in Tinder, but the chances are good that you underestimate just how distracted you are. The simple rule of thumb is that if your child is awake and active, your phone should be asleep. Once your child is napping or down for the night, then use social media or the Web to your heart's delight.

Of course, if one of the things you want to do on social media is post photos of your adorable infant sleeping or making adorable faces in the crib, you should do your best not to drop your smartphone or tablet on their little head. Parenting is guilt-inducing enough without actively hurting your child, particularly if the only reason is to gain a few more likes on Instagram.

Privacy

For expecting moms and dads, the most challenging cybertraps revolve around the issue of privacy. If you accept the definition of "privacy" as "the ability to control the collection, use, and distribution of personal information," the problems are immediately evident. It is difficult, if not impossible, to fully control the corporate and governmental collection of data about each one of us, even if we actively try to avoid such harvesting. The collection and analysis of personal data is embedded in virtually every aspect of our daily lives, and will only grow more so in the years to come.

That's particularly true in the case of pregnant women, who offer retailers and advertisers such a tempting economic target.

While it may not be possible to avoid all data collection, let alone control how it is used and re-distributed, that does not mean that we are required to feed the beast. If you are concerned about the rampant levels of data collection, then it is important to take some time to familiarize yourself with social media and app privacy policies. This is not the most enjoyable reading, needless to say, but it is really the only way to have some idea of what your period tracking or baby weight app is doing with your data. It may be that you and your partner will decide that the benefits outweigh the potential risks and that is certainly a legitimate decision; my recommendation is simply to have as much information as possible before you start recording what is often very personal data.

Although generally written in obtuse legalese, at least social media sites and apps typically have privacy policies that theoretically impose some limits on what they can do with the data they collect. That is NOT true for pretty much anyone who reads your posts or views the images you put online. Remember, "information wants to be free," and when you digitize anything — text, photos, videos — your ability to control its spread is inherently compromised. Once you post it online, have no illusions: there is no way to completely control what happens to it. Social media sites offer increasingly sophisticated privacy settings, but the protection they offer is illusory. If just one of your "friends' decides to do so, he or she can save or capture your content and redistribute it to the rest of the world.

Here's a good rule of thumb to keep in mind: if an online Web site or service needs privacy settings, that's a pretty good indication that it is not actually "private." Services like Dropbox or OneDrive, for instance, don't need privacy settings because they are password-protected. If you create a folder of child photos to share with your family, the only people who can view that folder are those to whom you purposely give permission. That is still not a guarantee that your child's photo will stay off the Web, but it does limit the potential number of suspects.

Identity, Narcissism, and Empathy

Many of the cybertraps that I've discussed in this book are immediately obvious. If you get into an accident with your child while texting, or if you drop your smartphone on his head, the connection between your misuse of a digital and effect is painfully clear.

However, one of the things that is so daunting about parenting is that the consequences of your decisions, many of which are made in a sleep-deprived fog and by themselves are utterly unremarkable, will not be known for months or years. That is unfortunately true for many if not most of the cybertraps I've discussed in this book. Are there adverse medical consequences arising out of the use of digital devices? Are we reducing the level of empathy in our society? Are text messages and instant messaging destroying the English language? If your child starts using a tablet at 10 months, will he or she wind up near-sighted or lack the ability to focus on tasks? These are legitimate questions, but ones that will take years to answer.

One activity that straddles both categories is the posting of updates, images, and videos of your children on social media. There is a very small but non-zero chance that your child will suffer some headline-grabbing harm as a result. Fortunately, however, the reality is that the odds are greater on any given day that you will drop your iPhone on your child.

The less visibly and immediately harmful consequences of posting about your child on social media have to do with identity. Thanks in large part to the enormous reach and global popularity of social media, this may be one of the most dynamic and fluid times for the formation of personal identity in human history. As your child grows up and slowly enters the online world (as slowly as possible!), he or she will naturally want as much freedom to establish an identity as possible. Every photo and video you post is an incremental infringement on his or her ability to do so. In a relative short period of time, I predict that this will be seen as a lesser human rights issue.

Even if you believe that there are benefits that outweigh the potential impact on your child, you should think about the example you are setting for your child. Researchers are already discovering that an increase in narcissism is one of the toxic byproducts of our digital age. If our children grows up with the experience of constantly being photographed and shared, it is likely that they will continue that behavior when they have their own social media accounts. Teens and tweens were self-absorbed long before Mark Zuckerberg launched Facebook; the last thing they need is any encouragement to engage in further self-indulgence.

It's not necessarily true that an increase in narcissism is directly matched by a corresponding decrease in empathy. In theory, someone could be an empathetic narcissist, I suppose. But in general, there does seem to be a pretty strong inverse correlation. Even if you are not concerned about raising a little narcissist, it is worth thinking carefully about the importance of encouraging your child to be empathetic. Not only is empathy an important quality for a child to have — it is valuable for relationships, school, jobs, *etc.* — but it is also a critically important social skill. A good argument can be made that empathy is what makes it possible for us to live together at all.

A single social media post of a birth announcement or even the occasional birthday photo is not going to destroy your child's empathy nor crush his or her emerging identity. The attitudes and behaviors of our children are inculcated over months and years, not days. Our goal as parents should be to set the best example possible and to create the opportunity for them to develop their best selves. Above all, that requires a thoughtful and proactive approach to the use of technology in parenting.

Ironically, it may be that a decision to delay the use of technology may well become a competitive advantage for your child in our technology-saturated world. *In regione caecorum rex est luscus* ("In the land of the blind, the one-eyed man is king").

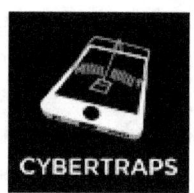

Connect With Frederick Lane Online

Thank you for purchasing this e-book and for taking the time to read it. If you found this book to be interesting, useful, shocking, alarming, accessible, charming and witty—please leave a review for me on Amazon at *Cybertraps for Expecting Moms & Dads*

If you'd like to keep up to date on my latest books, news, and the latest Cybertraps, please join my mailing list.

If you have any suggestions for ways it can be improved or additional resources that should be added, or if you just want to reach out, you can find me online everywhere:

Via Email: FSLane3@gmail.com

On LinkedIn: Frederick Lane

On Facebook: Fred Lane

On Twitter: @Cybertraps

At FrederickLane.com

Word of mouth is a huge help in promoting any book or product. If you found this book useful and informative, please tell your friends and acquaintances about it on your various social networks or by email.

Thank you!!

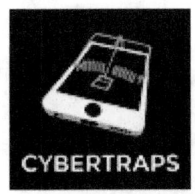

Appendix A

Drafting a Digital Technology Plan
for Pregnancy and Infancy

Digital technology and social media already touch on just about every aspect of pregnancy and parenting and there is little chance that will change. If anything, current trends suggest that technology will be increasingly important factor in every single aspect of our lives. In order to better protect the safety, health, privacy, and identity of yourselves and your child, you should think about and discuss your answers to the following questions. Where appropriate, it may be helpful to write down your responses in the form of a simple agreement between the two of you about how you will use digital technology and social media during the course of your pregnancy and in raising your child.

Obviously, this is a lot of things to think about, so you probably will want to space it out over several different conversations. Just try to think of these questions as "Cards for the Perpetuation of Humanity."

Q. Do you routinely carry your cell phone in your front pocket, or in a purse or bag that hangs near your waist?

Q. Do you routinely use your laptop on your lap?

Q. Have you had a fertility test or discussed the possible impact of technology on your fertility with a health care provider?

Q. Do you use your cell phone while driving?

Q. Do you use your cell phone while walking

Q. Do you take a lot of selfies? Do you take selfies in dangerous or risky locations?

Q. Do you using dating Web sites or geo-social dating apps? If so, which ones?

Q. Is your relationship with your co-parent or prospective co-parent monogamous?

Q. Are you suffering from any sexually transmitted infections (STIs)? Have you been tested for STIs recently?

Q. Do you feel that your partner's digital device habits interfere with your relationship? In what ways? What guidelines regarding device use would make you feel more connected?

Q. Do you feel that digital devices are interfering with your sleep or your partner's sleep?

Q. Do you feel that digital devices are interfering with your sex life?

Q. Do you use sex toys (including digital devices) that have active Bluetooth or WiFi connections? Do you ever fall asleep with those devices on your bed?

Q. How secure is the data collected (if any) by the sex toys or sex apps you use?

Q. Do you use one or more sex toys that can be controlled remotely over the Internet? Has the manufacturer taken steps to prevent hacking?

Q. Do one or both of you use pornography as a sexual or masturbatory aid? Do either of you feel that pornography interferes with your sexual relationship?

Q. Do you use one or more devices to monitor your daily activity, including exercise and/or heart rate? Are you comfortable with the possibility that it could alert the manufacturer to a pregnancy before you know yourself?

Q. Are you using or do you plan to use a smartphone app to track your period, days of optimum conception, etc.? Have you read the software publisher's privacy policy, particularly with respect to data collection and data sharing?

Q. What social media guidelines do you and your partner feel are appropriate regarding pregnancy announcements? Who should be told, in what order, and how?

Q. Do you have any family members or friends who have had a difficult time conceiving? What steps, if any, should you take to protect or be considerate of their feelings?

Q. Do you feel it is appropriate to post a photo or video of your home pregnancy test or of the results?

Q. Do you feel it is appropriate to use software to manipulate a photo of your pregnancy test in an effort to determine results as soon as possible? Are you comfortable asking someone online to assist you in doing so?

Q. How often do you research medical information on the Internet? How often do you rely on the information you find?

Q. What changes, if any, will you make in your use of digital devices during pregnancy?

Q. During your pregnancy, do you use (or do you plan to use) your cell phone while driving or walking?

Q. What steps will you take (if any) to minimize the impact of noise or heat from digital devices on your fetus?

Q. What steps will you take (if any) to minimize the exposure of your fetus to various forms of radiation, including radio-frequency, WiFi, and Bluetooth?

Q. Will it bother you to receive pregnancy-related advertisements and offers during the course of your pregnancy? What steps are you willing to take to reduce the amount of personal data collected by businesses, advertisers, and other organizations?

Q. How many advertising-supported Web sites or apps are you using (or plan to use) during your pregnancy? Have you read the privacy policies for those Web sites and/or apps?

Q. Do you and/or your partner plan to post photos during the course of pregnancy? Which social media channels will be used? Do you both have to agree before a particular image or video is uploaded to the Web?

Q. Would it bother one or both of you to learn that photo(s) of your baby bump have been copied and uploaded to pregnancy fetish Web sites? What steps, if any, have you and your partner taken to reduce the chances of that happening?

Q. If you do post pregnancy-related photos of yourself on social media, are you prepared to deal with the comments, critiques, and criticisms of your weight, the size of your bump, your eating habits, and your fashion sense?

Q. Do you and/or your partner plan to post a sonogram of your fetus on social media? Have you removed any personal or private information that may be printed on the sonogram?

Q. Do you plan to ask family, friends, or complete strangers to offer opinions about the sex of your child based on his or her sonogram?

Q. Do you or your partner think that the privacy interests of your unborn child should be taken into account when posting sonogram?

Q. Do you and your partner want a visual record of your child's birth?

Q. Do you want information posted to social media (Facebook, Twitter, Instagram, *etc.*) during labor or while the birth is occurring?

Q. Do you want photos, video, or both?

Q. Will one of you record the event or do you plan to hire a professional?

Q. Have you reviewed the policy of your birthing facility regarding photos and videos during birth?

Q. If no media policy exists, have you discussed photos and videos with your physician or midwife? Have you obtained the consent of each person who will be in the room with you?

Q. Do you plan to post updates, photos, or videos online? During the birth or afterwards?

Q. Do you and your partner want to broadcast the birth live on social media? Have you reviewed the terms of service for whichever social media service you plan to use? Do you and your partner understand your digital technology and social media well enough to avoid broadcasting by accident?

Q. Do you plan to send out a birth announcement for your new child? If so, will you send it through the mail, electronically, or some combination of the two?

Q. If you decide to send announcement, what information will you and your partner include?

Q. What are the main factors for you and your partner in selecting a name for your child?

Q. Are there any family members or friends who should be told about your child's birth before a public announcement is made?

Q. Do you have any interest in asking the Internet to name your child?

Q. Do you or your partner think that it is important to reserve domain names, email addresses, or social media accounts in the name of your child? Would one or both of you be willing to change the spelling of your child's name to make it easier to reserve digital real estate?

Q. Have you and your partner thought about or discussed when your new child will be first allowed to use social media? What are the guidelines that you think should be enforced?

Q. Do you and your partner believe that you have the right to post about your child on social media (including text, photos, and/or video) until he or she is old enough to object?

Q. Do you and your partner think that your right to post about your child overrides his or her objections until he or she is 18? If not, at what point would you begin to respect your child's wishes?

Q. In particular, what rules should you and your partner establish regarding the posting of information and images of your child?

Q. More broadly, what rules will you and your partner have for yourselves regarding the use of technology while your child is present?

Q. Should you and your partner create a family contract regarding the use of technology, both for yourselves and for your child?

Q. How much would it bother you and/or your partner if your child's photo were used without your permission to create an Internet meme?

Q. How much would it bother you and/or your partner if your child's photo were used without your permission for advertising? Would you reaction depend upon the specific product or service for which it was being used?

Q. How much would it bother you and/or your partner if your child's photo were used without your permission by someone pretending to be the parent of your child?

Q. How much would it bother you and/or your partner if your child's photo were used without your permission for the sexual titillation or gratification of strangers?

Q. Do you and/or your partner know how to remove identifying information (particularly GPS location data) from photographs before posting them to social media?

Q. What would your reaction be if your child someday decide to sue you and/or your partner for posting information or images of him or her on social media without consent?

Q. How important is it to you and/or your partner to record data about various aspects of your child's health and development?

Q. If you buy "smart" equipment for your baby or use a data-tracking app, will you and/or your partner read the manufacturer's privacy policy, particularly with respect to the sharing of that data?

Q. How comfortable are you and/or partner with purchasing and using devices around your newborn that require the use of Bluetooth and WiFi in order to function properly?

Q. Are you and/or your partner comfortable using the growing number of devices that listen to your conversations with your child and transmit them to the Web for various types of analysis?

Q. How will you and/or your partner avoid paying more attention to the data demands of "smart" devices and apps than to your child?

Q. Do you and/or your partner know what steps are necessary to secure any devices that are connected to the Internet (particularly baby monitors)?

Q. What rules do you and/or your partner want to have regarding the use of digital devices around your child?

Q. What rules do you and/or your partner want to have regarding the use of digital devices while transporting your child in a car, in a stroller, or in a sling (or similar carrier)?

Q. Do you think that it is appropriate to use a digital device (or a television or book) while feeding your newborn?

Q. Have you discussed with your pediatrician the possible risks of Bluetooth or WiFi radiation for your newborn?

Q. Have you discussed with your pediatrician or optometrist the possible impact of digital devices on your infant's vision?

Q. How early do you and your partner think your child should be allowed to use an electronic device (smartphone, tablet, toy, *etc.*)?

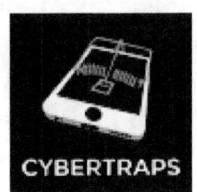

Acknowledgments

Coincidentally, my wife Amy is writing the acknowledgments for her forthcoming book, *Lust on Trial: American Art, Law, and Culture During the Reign of Anthony Comstock,* which will be published in 2017 by Columbia University Press. I am pleased to say that I have a place in those acknowledgments, much as she does in these. It is a rare privilege to have a partner capable of providing such helpful editorial feedback and criticism. This is a better book than it would have been without her assistance. Much the same can be said about life as whole.

As always, my family has been a source of inspiration. Our four boys — Ben, Graham, Peter, and Emmett — have provided endless opportunities to discover the benefits and challenges that technology presents for parents. As they have gotten older, all have contributed in various ways to my book projects, including this one, and I am grateful for their assistance. They appear to be navigating the transition from adolescence to adulthood with grace and dignity in this technology-infused world and that is, I think, about as much as one can ask. And of course, my ongoing love and affection for my siblings Jon, Elizabeth, and Kate, their spouses and children, and my parents, Warren and Anne Lane. My mother in particular is thankful she didn't have to deal with the technology-related topics I discuss in this book.

As I noted in the introduction, this book arose out of a series of conversations with my then-upstairs neighbor Tami Mnoian. I am grateful for her suggestion and her encouragement over the course of this project.

As this project was getting under way, I had the good fortune to collaborate with a remarkable group of technology and educational specialists; together, we formed a non-profit group called the Coalition for Digital Educators, which will have its formal launch a few weeks from now. My sincere thanks to Alan Katzman for taking the lead in its formation, and to my fellow founding members, Meagan Davis, Denise DeRosa, Diana Graber, Janelle Maitland, and Liz Repking. Particular thanks is due to Janelle and Denise for offering feedback on early chapters in the manuscript.

One of the pleasures of working on the Cybertraps series has been the opportunity to interview different people about their expertise and experiences. My thanks to Ramin Bastani, Jonathan Plotzger, Zhenya Pozharny, and Benton Lane for taking the time to answer my questions and for their thoughtful perspectives. I look forward to adding additional voices to this book as I update it in the months to come.

I would like to extend particular thanks to Andrea B. Goetz, the Assistant Commissioner for the Office of Clinical Practice, Policy & Support for the New York City Administration for Children's Services. She was kind enough to invite me to participate via Skype in a wonderful panel discussion on June 24, 2016 about the impact of social media on vulnerable youth. The event tied in nicely with the themes of this book, and I look forward to working further with Andrea and her colleagues on these issues. I would also like to acknowledge CNN's Kelly Wallace for her excellent work as moderator of the panel and her ongoing reporting on parenting and child-related topics.

Once again, Colin Gliech demonstrated his terrific creativity in the design of the cover for this book. Over the course of a long, intense summer of writing, I would periodically look at the cover and be reminded that it deserved to have text behind it. You may not be able to tell a book by its cover, but I hope that my text does justice to Colin's work.

Throughout the course of this project, a number of people have offered encouragement and occasional links to relevant articles. I would particularly like to thank Troy Hutchings, Glenn Lipson, Sam Albert, Pat Vogelpohl for their interest and their input.

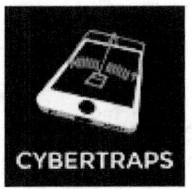

Endnotes

Endnotes for the Introduction

I.1 In recent years, many medical and public health professionals have started using the phrase "sexually transmitted infection" in place of the more well-known "sexually transmitted disease" (STD). The reason for the change, according to the American Sexual Health Association, is to better acknowledge that an individual may be infected through sexual contact but not fall sick or display any obvious symptoms of a "disease." "STDS/STIS," American Sexual Health Association, [n.d.] [last accessed on 16 June 2016 at http://www.ashasexualhealth.org/stdsstis/]. I will use the phrase "sexually transmitted infection" throughout this book, except when quoting someone directly.

Endnotes for Chapter One

1.1 It is fair to point out, of course, that some believe that it is possible to have too much of a good thing. For instance, midwives frequently argue that much of the technology used during labor is unnecessary, overly expensive, and possibly harmful (at least emotionally if not physically). *See, e.g.,* Marsden Wagner, MD, "Technology in Birth: First Do No Harm," Midwifery Today, 2000 [last accessed on 22 June 2016 at https://www.midwiferytoday.com/articles/technologyinbirth.asp].

1.2 Sara J. Martinez, "How the iPod and Other Audio Devices Are Destroying Your Ears," *The Atlantic*, December 15, 2011 [last accessed on 23 June 2016 at http://www.theatlantic.com/health/archive/2011/12/how-the-ipod-and-other-audio-devices-are-destroying-your-ears/249521/].

1.3 *See, e.g.,* "Environmental Issues," The Carnegie Cyber Academy, [n.d.] [last accessed on 23 June 2016 at http://www.carnegiecyberacademy.com/facultyPages/environment/issues.h Jane Wakefield, "Apple, Samsung and Sony face child labour claims," BBC News, January 19, 2016 [last accessed on 23 June 2016 at http://www.bbc.com/news/technology-35311456].

1.4 "Cell Phone Subscribers in the U.S., 1985–2010," InfoPlease.com, [n.d.] (quoting CTIA — The Wireless Association) [last accessed on 22 June 2016 at http://www.infoplease.com/ipa/A0933563.html.].

1.5 "Number of mobile phone users in the U.S. from 2012 to 2019 (in millions)," Statista, 2016 [last accessed on 22 June 2016 at http://www.statista.com/statistics/222306/forecast-of-smartphone-users-in-the-us/].

1.6 "Number of smartphone users in the United States from 2010 to 2019 (in millions)*," Statista, 2016 [last accessed on 22 June 2016 at http://www.statista.com/statistics/201182/forecast-of-smartphone-users-in-the-us/].

1.7 "Always Connected: How Smartphones and Social Keep Us Engaged," IDC, March 2013 [last accessed on 23 June 2016 at http://www.fredericklane.com/wp-content/uploads/2016/06/2013-IDC_Facebook_Always-Connected.pdf].

1.8 *Id.*

1.9 Lee Rainie and Kathryn Zickuhr, "Chapter One: Always on Connectivity," from Pew Research Center's "Americans'Views on Mobile Etiquette," August 26, 2015 [last accessed on 23 June 2016 at http://www.pewinternet.org/2015/08/26/chapter-1-always-on-connectivity/].

1.10 "Cellular Phones," American Cancer Society, [n.d.] [last accessed on 23 June 2016 at http://www.cancer.org/cancer/cancercauses/othercarcinogens/athome/cellu phones].

1.11 "SAR Values," S21, March 12, 2016 [last accessed on 25 June 2016 at http://www.s21.com/sar.htm. The article also has one of the more comprehensive listings of the SAR values for the leading models of cell phones.

1.12 "Microwaves, Radio Waves, and Other Types of Radiofrequency Radiation," American Cancer Society, May 31, 2016 [last accessed on 25 June 2016 at http://www.cancer.org/cancer/cancercauses/radiationexposureandcancer/ra radiation].

1.13 Moulder JE, Erdreich LS, Malyapa RS, Merritt J, Pickard WF, Vijayalaxmi, "Cell phones and cancer: what is the evidence for a connection?" *Radiation Research*, May 1999 [last accessed on 25 June 2016 at http://www.ncbi.nlm.nih.gov/pubmed/10319725].

1.14 Simon Chapman, Lamiae Azizi, Qingwei Luo, Freddy Sitas, "Has the incidence of brain cancer risen in Australia since the introduction of mobile phones 29 years ago?" *Cancer Epidemiology*, June 2016 [last accessed on 25 June 2016 at http://www.cancerepidemiology.net/article/S1877-7821(16)30050-

9/abstract].

1.15 Ally Fogg, "Men don't worry about their sperm count – but they should," *The Guardian*, March 31, 2015 [last accessed on 25 June 2016 at https://www.theguardian.com/commentisfree/2015/mar/31/sperm-count-worry-male-fertility-crisis].

1.16 Victoria Georgoff, "Do Cell Phones Harm Female Fertility?" *Parenting*, April 2, 2014 [last accessed on 25 June 2016 at http://www.parenting.com/fertility/infertility/do-cell-phones-harm-female-fertility].

1.17 John G. West, Nimmi S. Kapoor, Shu-Yuan Liao, June W. Chen, Lisa Bailey, and Robert A. Nagourney, "Multifocal Breast Cancer in Young Women with Prolonged Contact between Their Breasts and Their Cellular Phones," *Case Reports in Medicine*, 2013 [last accessed on 25 June 2016 at http://www.hindawi.com/journals/crim/2013/354682/].

1.18 Katharine Gammon, "Sperm Quality & Quantity Declining, Mounting Evidence Suggests," Live Science, August 28, 2012 [last accessed on 25 June 2016 at http://www.livescience.com/22694-global-sperm-count-decline.html].

1.19 Edmund Saunders, "Israel sperm banks find quality is plummeting," *Los Angeles Times*, August 15, 2012 [last accessed on 25 June 2016 at http://articles.latimes.com/2012/aug/15/world/la-fg-israel-sperm-20120816].

1.20 Jeremy Laurence, "Scientists warn of sperm count crisis," *Independent*, December 5, 2012 [last accessed on 25 June 2016 at http://www.independent.co.uk/news/science/scientists-warn-of-sperm-count-crisis-8382449.html].

1.21 Joe Millis, "Sperm count: Fertility in men on the decline due to everyday plastics say scientists," *International Business Times*, June 18, 2015 [last accessed on 26 June 2016 at http://www.ibtimes.co.uk/sperm-count-fertility-men-decline-due-everyday-plastics-say-scientists-1506746].

1.22 Caroline Ryan, "Mobiles 'could cut male fertility,'" BBC News, June 27, 2004 [last accessed on 26 June 2016 at http://news.bbc.co.uk/2/hi/health/3844871.stm].

1.23 Caroline McCarthy, "Chat on cell phone, become infertile?" c|net, October 24, 2006 [last accessed on 26 June 2016 at http://www.cnet.com/news/chat-on-cell-phone-become-infertile/; Tara Parker-Pope, "Good Question: Do Cellphones Affect Fertility?" *New York*

Times, February 19, 2008 [last accessed on 26 June 2016 at http://well.blogs.nytimes.com/2008/02/19/the-inbox-cell-phones-and-sperm/; "Talking on a mobile phone 'may lower male fertility,'" *Daily Mail*, May 20, 2011 [last accessed on 26 June 2016 at http://www.dailymail.co.uk/health/article-1389043/Family-planning-Mobile-phone-use-lower-male-fertility.html; Kelly Dickerson, "Cellphone Radiation Might Be a Drag on Sperm," livescience.com, June 11, 2014 [last accessed on 26 June 2016 at http://www.livescience.com/46273-cellphone-radiation-sperm-quality.html; "Mobile phones are 'cooking' men's sperm," *The Telegraph*, February 22, 2016 [last accessed on 26 June 2016 at http://www.telegraph.co.uk/news/health/news/12167957/Mobile-phones-are-cooking-mens-sperm.html].

1.24 Libby Clark, "Safeguard Your Sperm," *Men's Health*, October 5, 2010 [last accessed on 26 June 2016 at http://www.menshealth.com/health/the-effect-of-heat-on-sperm-production].

1.25 Orac, "No, cell phones are not 'cooking men''s sperm,'" ScienceBlogs, February 24, 2016 [last accessed on 26 June 2016 at http://scienceblogs.com/insolence/2016/02/24/no-cell-phones-are-not-cooking-mens-sperm/].

1.26 Frederik Joelving, "Is your laptop cooking your testicles?" Reuters, November 8, 2010 [last accessed on 17 July 2016 at http://www.reuters.com/article/us-laptop-testicles-idUSTRE6A457320101108].

1.27 *Id.*

Endnotes for Chapter Two

2.1 Thanks to various medical advances, of course, death is no longer the absolute barrier to reproduction that it once was. For the past sixty years or so, scientists have been able to successfully impregnate women using frozen sperm. Many women have given birth to children using sperm frozen prior to the death of their husband. *See, e.g.*, Amanda Ward, "The women who gave birth to their dead husbands' babies," *Daily Mail*, April 2, 2002 [last accessed on 19 June 2016 at http://www.dailymail.co.uk/health/article-107698/The-women-gave-birth-dead-husbands-babies.html]. There is also a growing trend of "post-mortem sperm retrieval," a request typically made when a man dies in a sudden accident or unexpected illness. "Making Babies After Death: It's Possible, But Is It Ethical?" Red Ice TV, June 13, 2013 [last accessed on 19 June 2016 at https://redice.tv/news/making-babies-after-death-it-s-possible-but-is-it-ethical; Steven Trask, "Woman wins permission to remove her dead partner's testicles in the hope of using his sperm to get pregnant," *Daily Mail*, May 27, 2016 [last accessed on 28 June 2016 at http://www.dailymail.co.uk/news/article-3612178/Woman-wins-permission-remove-dead-partner-s-testicles.html]. One woman even launched a legal battle to use her deceased daughter's frozen eggs and donated sperm to give birth to her own granddaughter. Jo MacFarlane and Stephen Adams, "British mum, 59, in bid for world medical first: I'll give birth to baby of my dead daughter," *Daily Mail*, February 21, 2015 [last accessed on 28 June 2016 at http://www.dailymail.co.uk/news/article-2963277/British-mum-59-bid-world-medical-ll-birth-baby-dead-daughter.html]. All such procedures raise significant social and ethical issues.

2.2 Maggie Fox, "Talking to death: texts, phones kill 16,000: study," Reuters, September 23, 2010 [last accessed on 19 June 2016 at http://www.reuters.com/article/us-cellphones-driving-idUSTRE68M53K20100923].

2.3 David L. Strayer, Frank A. Drews, and Dennis J. Crouch, "A Comparison of the Cell Phone Driver and the Drunk Driver," *Human Factors*, Summer 2006 [last accessed on 28 June 2016 at http://www.distraction.gov/downloads/pdfs/a-comparison-of-the-cell-phone-driver-and-the-drunk-driver.pdf].

2.4 Christopher Woody, "Cell phones are causing more and more car crashes," *Business Insider*, May 31, 2015 [last accessed on 19 June 2016 at http://www.businessinsider.com/cell-phones-causing-car-crashes-and-deaths-2015-5]. The Council did not estimate the number of injuries or deaths that resulted from the accidents.

2.5 Michael Austin, "Texting While Driving: How Dangerous is it?" *Car & Driver*, June 2009 [last accessed on 28 June 2016 at http://www.caranddriver.com/features/texting-while-driving-how-dangerous-is-it].

2.6 *Id.*

2.7 Erin Dooley, "Distracted Walking: How 'Petextrians' Are Endangering Our Streets," August 10, 2015 [last accessed on 19 June

2016 at http://abcnews.go.com/US/distracted-walking-petextrians-endangering-streets/story?id=32990067].

2.8 *Id.*

2.9 Marcene Robinson, "Think it's safe to type a quick text while walking? Guess again," *UB Reporter*, February 13, 2014 [last accessed on 28 June 2016 at https://www.buffalo.edu/ubreporter/research/news.host.html/content/shared/reporter-articles/stories/2014/February/texting_walking.detail.html].

2.10 Caitlin McCormack, "Distracted Walking a Major Pedestrian Safety Concern," SafeSoundFamily.com, February 23, 2016 [last accessed on 28 June 2016 at http://safesoundfamily.com/blog/distracted-walking-a-major-pedestrian-safety-concern/].

2.11 "Take Steps to Avoid Injury or Death While Walking," National Safety Council, [n.d.] [last accessed on 28 June 2016 at http://www.nsc.org/learn/safety-knowledge/Pages/news-and-resources-pedestrian-safety.aspx].

2.12 Erin Dooley, "Distracted Walking: How 'Petextrians' Are Endangering Our Streets," August 10, 2015 [last accessed on 19 June 2016 at http://abcnews.go.com/US/distracted-walking-petextrians-endangering-streets/story?id=32990067].

2.13 Janek Schmidt, "Always practise safe text: the German traffic light for smartphone zombies," *The Guardian*, April 29, 2016 [last accessed on 28 June 2016 at https://www.theguardian.com/cities/2016/apr/29/always-practise-safe-text-the-german-traffic-light-for-smartphone-zombies].

2.14 "'Pokemon Go' is afflicting players with real-world injuries," *New York Post*, July 9, 2016 [last accessed on 09 July 2016 at http://nypost.com/2016/07/09/pokemon-go-is-afflicting-players-with-real-world-injuries/].

2.15 Cristina Quinn, "Texting While Walking Draws Safety Concerns — and an App," WGBH, December 20, 2011 [last accessed on 28 June 2016 at http://www.wgbh.org/articles/Texting-While-Walking-Draws-Safety-Concerns-mdash-And-An-App-5140]; "Manitoba researchers eye walking-texting safety app," CBC News, September 5, 2013 [last accessed on 28 June 2016 at http://www.cbc.ca/news/canada/manitoba/manitoba-researchers-eye-walking-texting-safety-app-1.1319784]; "New app aims to keep people safe while texting and walking," *NY Daily News,* March 10, 2014 [last accessed on 28 June 2016 at http://www.nydailynews.com/life-style/app-people-walk-text-article-1.1716525].

2.16 Narcissism, *Cambridge Dictionaries Online*, [n.d.] [last accessed on 29 June 2016 at http://dictionary.cambridge.org/dictionary/english/narcissism].

2.17 "Narcissistic Personality Disorder — Definition," Mayo Clinic, November 18, 2014 [last accessed on 29 June 2016 at http://www.mayoclinic.org/diseases-conditions/narcissistic-personality-disorder/basics/definition/con-20025568].

2.18 Arthur C. Brooks, "Narcissism Is Increasing. So You're Not That Special," *New York Times*, February 13, 2016 [last accessed on 29 June 2016 at http://www.nytimes.com/2016/02/14/opinion/narcissism-is-increasing-so-youre-not-so-special.html].

2.19 Lisa Firestone, Ph.D., "Is Social Media to Blame For the Rise In Narcissism?" *Psychology Today*, November 29, 2012 [last accessed on 29 June 2016 at https://www.psychologytoday.com/blog/compassion-matters/201211/is-social-media-blame-the-rise-in-narcissism].

2.20 Meehan, Sean Ross, *Mediating American Autobiography: Photography in Emerson, Thoreau, Douglass, and Whitman,* University of Missouri Press (2008), p. 24 [ISBN 978-0-8262-6640-8] [last accessed on 29 June 2016 at https://books.google.com/books?id=Q8Lc2WJankUC&pg=PA23].

2.21 Jon Wurtzel, "Taking Pictures with Your Phone," BBC News, September 18, 2001 [last accessed on 29 June 2016 at http://news.bbc.co.uk/2/hi/science/nature/1550622.stm]. Prior to that, photographers would take photos with their digital cameras, download them to a computer, and then upload them to a Web site or email them to friends.

2.22 Tomi T. Ahonen, "Camera Stats: World has 5.8B Cameras by 4B Unique Camera Owners: 89% of camera owners use a cameraphone to take pictures; This year first time 1 Trillion pictures are taken," Communities Dominate Brands, August 11, 2014 [last accessed on 29 June 2016 at http://communities-dominate.blogs.com/brands/2014/08/camera-stats-world-has-48b-cameras-by-4b-unique-camera-owners-88-of-them-use-cameraphone-to-take-pic.html].

2.23 Paul Malcore, "Selfie Obsession: The Rise of Social Media Narcissism," Rawhide.org, December 29, 2015 [last accessed on 29 June

2016 at http://www.rawhide.org/blog/infographics/selfie-obsession-the-rise-of-social-media-narcissism/].

2.24 Jonathan Perlman, "Australian man 'invented the selfie after drunken night out,'" *The Telegraph*, November 19, 2013 [last accessed on 29 June 2016 at http://www.telegraph.co.uk/news/worldnews/australiaandthepacific/austral man-invented-the-selfie-after-drunken-night-out.html]. Hope later told the Australian Broadcasting Company that he hadn't actually coined the word, which he said was in common usage in his area at the time of his accident. Ben Zimmer, "No, a Drunken Australian Man Did Not Coin the Word Selfie," Slate.com, November 22, 2013 [last accessed on 29 June 2016 at http://www.slate.com/blogs/lexicon_valley/2013/11/22/selfie_etymology_a].

2.25 Sarah Graham, "Take a lot of selfies? Then you may be MENTALLY ILL: Two thirds of patients with body image disorders obsessively take photos of themselves," *Daily Mail*, April 10, 2014 [last accessed on 29 June 2016 at http://www.dailymail.co.uk/sciencetech/article-2601606/Take-lot-selfies-Then-MENTALLY-ILL-Two-thirds-patients-body-image-disorders-obsessively-photos-themselves.html].

2.26 Zoe Williams, "Me! Me! Me! Are we living through a narcissism epidemic?" *The Guardian*, March 2, 2016 [last accessed on 29 June 2016 at https://www.theguardian.com/lifeandstyle/2016/mar/02/narcissism-epidemic-self-obsession-attention-seeking-oversharing].

2.27 Zachary Crockett, "The Tragic Data Behind Selfie Fatalities," Priceonomics.com, January 29, 2016 [last accessed on 29 June 2016 at http://priceonomics.com/the-tragic-data-behind-selfie-fatalities/].

2.28 Mark Piggott, "Selfie dangers: Teen falls 9 floors to his death as he poses on rooftop in Russia," *International Business Times*, September 30, 2015 [last accessed on 30 June 2016 at http://www.ibtimes.co.uk/selfie-dangers-teen-falls-9-floors-his-death-he-poses-rooftop-russia-1521743].

2.29 Chris Matyszczyk, "Russian government issues guide to avoiding hazardous selfies," c|net, July 7, 2015 [last accessed on 30 June 2016 at http://www.cnet.com/news/russian-government-issues-guide-to-avoiding-hazardous-selfies/].

2.30 Qin Xie, "Is this the most dangerous selfie spot in the world? Tourists perch on 2,769ft high cliff in Brazil to get the perfect shot," *Daily*

Mail, April 20, 2016 [last accessed on 30 June 2016 at http://www.dailymail.co.uk/travel/travel_news/article-3546181/The-new-nail-biting-craze-Brazil-Hanging-edge-2-769-foot-cliff-face-perfect-shot.html].

2.31 Hugh Morris, "Trolltunga death an accident waiting to happen, says tour guide," *The Telegraph*, September 10, 2015 [last accessed on 30 June 2016 at http://www.telegraph.co.uk/travel/news/Trolltunga-death-an-accident-waiting-to-happen-says-tour-guide/].

2.32 *Id.*, quoting *The Telegraph* reporter Meabh Ritchie.

2.33 *Id.*

Endnotes for Chapter Three

3.1 "Top Gun (1986) — Quotes," Internet Movie Data Base, [n.d.] [last accessed on 11 June 2016 at http://www.imdb.com/title/tt0092099/quotes.]

3.2 Many argue that geo-social dating apps have little if anything to do with "dating" as that term is traditionally understood, since these apps are designed to reduce complicated "compatibility" algorithms to the two most primal factors in human interaction: physical proximity AND horniness. Others claim that the success of geo-social apps (and in particular, Tinder) stems from the fact that compatibility tests are a crock and that at least in terms of first impressions, the only thing that matters is a person's appearance. *See, e.g.*, Nick Bilton, "Tinder, the Fast-Growing Dating App, Taps an Age Old Truth," *The New York Times*, October 29, 2014 [last accessed on 11 June 2016 at http://www.nytimes.com/2014/10/30/fashion/tinder-the-fast-growing-dating-app-taps-an-age-old-truth.html].

3.3 T.J. Matthews, "Operation Match," *The Harvard Crimson*, November 3, 1965 [last accessed on 21 February 2015 at http://www.thecrimson.com/article/1965/11/3/operation-match-pif-you-stop-to/]; David Leonhardt, "The Famous Founder of Operation Match," *The New York Times*, March 28, 2006 [last accessed on 21 February 2016 at http://www.nytimes.com/2006/03/28/business/29leonside.html]. Fun historical fact: Daniel Ginsburg used proceeds from the sale of his share of Compatibility Research to finish his education and wound up as a professor of law at Harvard Law School. He was appointed by President

Reagan to the U.S. Court of Appeals for the District of Columbia in 1986, and was nominated to the U.S. Supreme Court in 1987 following the defeat of Robert Bork's nomination. It was revealed, however, that he had smoked marijuana with students while teaching at Harvard and he withdrew his nomination. The vacancy was filled by Anthony Kennedy in the spring of 1988.

3.4 "One-third of married couples in U.S. meet online: study," *New York Daily News*, June 4, 2013 [last accessed on 17 June 2016 at http://www.nydailynews.com/life-style/one-third-u-s-marriages-start-online-dating-study-article-1.1362743].

3.5 Patrick Strudwick, "Grindr founder Joel Simkhai: 'I've found love on my dating app - and my mum keeps trying to hook me up!', *The Independent*, July 9, 2014 [last accessed on 10 June 2016 at http://www.independent.co.uk/life-style/gadgets-and-tech/features/grindr-founder-joel-simkhai-ive-found-love-on-my-dating-app-and-my-mum-keeps-trying-to-hook-me-up-9596054.html].

3.6 Intentionally or unintentionally, the Tinder programmers incorporated an ancient bias against the left and those who are left-handed into the operation of the app. *See, e.g.,* "How did 'sinister,' the Latin word for 'left-handed,' get its current meaning?", English Language & Usage, August 23, 2011 [last accessed on 10 June 2016 at http://english.stackexchange.com/questions/39092/how-did-sinister-the-latin-word-for-left-handed-get-its-current-meaning]. The Web site AnythingLeftHanded.co.uk has a list of other biases and superstitions about left-handers: http://www.anythinglefthanded.co.uk/being-lh/lh-info/myths.html [last accessed on 10 June 2016].

3.7 Issie Lapowsky, "How Tinder Is Winning the Mobile Dating Wars," *Inc.*, May 23, 2013 [last accessed on 17 June 2016 at http://www.inc.com/issie-lapowsky/how-tinder-is-winning-the-mobile-dating-wars.html].

3.8 "7th Annual Crunchies Awards," *TechCrunch*, February 10, 2014 [last accessed on 10 June 2016 at http://techcrunch.com/events/7th-annual-crunchies-awards/winners/].

3.9 Craig Smith, "By the Numbers: 41 Impressive tinder Statistics," DMR, May 29, 2016 [last accessed on 10 June 2016 at http://expandedramblings.com/index.php/tinder-statistics/].

3.10 *Id.*

3.11 Nancy Jo Sales, "Tinder and the Dawn of the 'Dating

Apocalypse,'" *Vanity Fair*, September 2015 [last accessed on 11 June 2016 at http://www.vanityfair.com/culture/2015/08/tinder-hook-up-culture-end-of-dating].

3.12 Amanda Marcotte, "Let's All Throw Ourselves Another Moral-Panic Party About Technology," *Slate*, August 6, 2015 [last accessed on 12 June 2016 at http://www.slate.com/blogs/xx_factor/2015/08/06/tinder_is_causing_a_dat].

3.13 Jesse Singal, "Has Tinder Really Sparked a Dating Apocalypse?" *New York Magazine*, August 12, 2015 [last accessed on 12 June 2016 at http://nymag.com/scienceofus/2015/08/has-tinder-really-sparked-a-dating-apocalypse.html].

3.14 Karen Kaplan, "The paradox of millennial sex: More casual hookups, fewer partners," *Los Angeles Times*, May 9, 2015 [last accessed on 12 June 2016 at http://www.latimes.com/science/sciencenow/la-sci-sn-millennials-sex-attitudes-20150508-story.html]; Jean Twenge, Ryne Sherman, and Brooke E. Wells, "Changes in American Adults' Sexual Behavior and Attitudes, 1972-2012," *Archives of Sexual Behavior*, May 5, 2015 [available for purchase at http://link.springer.com/article/10.1007%2Fs10508-015-0540-2].

3.15 Sophie Jamieson, "Dr Lucy Worsley: dating apps like Tinder are destroying the art of romance," *The Telegraph*, October 6, 2016 [last accessed on 12 June 2016 at http://www.telegraph.co.uk/news/celebritynews/11915040/Dr-Lucy-Worsley-dating-apps-like-Tinder-are-destroying-the-art-of-romance.html].

3.16 *Id.*

3.17 Andrew L. Yarrow, "Falling Marriage Rates Reveal Economic Fault Lines," *New York Times*, February 6, 2015 [last accessed on 12 June 2016 at http://www.nytimes.com/2015/02/08/fashion/weddings/falling-marriage-rates-reveal-economic-fault-lines.html?_r=2&login=facebook].

3.18 Wendy Wong and Kim Parker, "Record Share of Americans Have Never Married," Pew Research Center, September 24, 2014 [last accessed on 30 June 2016 at http://www.pewsocialtrends.org/2014/09/24/record-share-of-americans-have-never-married/#will-todays-never-married-adults-eventually-marry].

3.19 Tom Keane, "Millennials, reject timely marriage at your own risk," *The Boston Globe*, July 27, 2014 [last accessed at http://www.bostonglobe.com/opinion/2014/07/27/millennials-reject-timely-marriage-your-own-risk/AgCRUNzxN07BOU4Gn2oISI/story.html].

3.20 Naomi Schaefer Riley, "Tinder is tearing society apart," *New York Post*, August 16, 2016 [last accessed on 15 July 2016 at http://nypost.com/2015/08/16/tinder-is-tearing-apart-society/].

3.21 Gabriela Barkho, "Why are millennials putting off marriage? Let me count the ways," *Washington Post*, June 6, 2016 [last accessed on 30 June 2016 at https://www.washingtonpost.com/news/soloish/wp/2016/06/06/why-are-millennials-putting-off-marriage-let-me-count-the-ways/].

3.22 Joyce A. Martin, M.P.H; Brady E. Hamilton, Ph.D.; and Michelle J.K. Osterman, M.H.S., "Births in the United States, 2013," NCHS Data Brief No. 175, December 2014 [last accessed on 12 June 2016 at http://www.cdc.gov/nchs/data/databriefs/db175.htm].

3.23 John Bingham, "How teenage pregnancy collapsed after birth of social media," *The Telegraph*, March 9, 2016 http://www.telegraph.co.uk/news/health/news/12189376/How-teenage-pregnancy-collapsed-after-birth-of-social-media.html].

3.24 Aziz Ansari, "Everything You Thought You Knew About L-O-V-E Is Wrong," *Time*, June 4, 2015 [last accessed on 15 July 2016 at http://time.com/aziz-ansari-modern-romance/]. It is worth noting that in January 2018, Ansari was the subject of a highly critical story on *Babe.net* that accused him of sexual misconduct during an encounter with an unnamed female photographer he met at an Emmy Awards after-party. Katie Way, "I went on a date with Aziz Ansari. It turned into the worst night of my life," *Babe.net*, January 13, 2018 [last accessed on 20 October 2018 at https://babe.net/2018/01/13/aziz-ansari-28355]. Ansari vigorously denied any wrongdoing; his statement was appended to the *Babe.net* story.

3.25 Megan Friedman, "Are Dating Apps Changing Marriage As We Know It?" *Redbook*, August 21, 2015 [last accessed on 30 June 2016 at http://www.redbookmag.com/love-sex/relationships/news/a39369/tinder-hinge-dating-apps-marriage-cheating/].

3.26 Steve Lohr, "For Impatient Web Users, an Eye Blink Is Just Too Long to Wait," *New York Times*, February 29, 2012 [last accessed on 15 July 2016 at http://www.nytimes.com/2012/03/01/technology/impatient-web-users-flee-slow-loading-sites.html].

Endnotes for Chapter Four

<u>4.1</u> Beymer, M.R.; Weiss, R.E.; Bolan, R.K.; Rudy, E.T.; Bourque, L.B.; Rodriguez, J.P.; and Morisky, D.E., "Sex on demand: geosocial networking phone apps and risk of sexually transmitted infections among a cross-sectional sample of men who have sex with men in Los Angeles County," *Sexually Transmitted Infections*, June 12, 2014 [last accessed on 13 June 2016 and available for purchase at http://sti.bmj.com/content/90/7/567.long].

<u>4.2</u> Rhode Island Department of Health, "HEALTH Releases New Data on Infectious Syphilis, Gonorrhea, and HIV," May 22, 2015 [last accessed on 13 June 2016 at http://www.ri.gov/press/view/24889].

<u>4.3</u> Marion Warnica, "Social media blamed for Alberta's gonorrhea and syphilis 'outbreak levels,'" CBC News, April 26, 2016 http://www.cbc.ca/news/canada/edmonton/social-media-blamed-for-alberta-s-gonorrhea-and-syphilis-outbreak-levels-1.3554228]. An inability to track down infectious individuals and their family members, friends, and sexual partners could have grave consequences in the event of a fast-moving diseases. For a dramatic and extremely well-written case study of how this worked in the early stages of the AIDS crisis, I highly recommend <u>*And the Band Played On*</u>, by Randy Shilts (St. Martin's Press, 1987).

<u>4.4</u> Rick Kelsey, "Dating apps increasing rates of sexually transmitted infections, say doctors," BBC Newsbeat, November 2, 2015 [last accessed on 9 July 2016 at http://www.bbc.co.uk/newsbeat/article/34008736/dating-apps-increasing-rates-of-sexually-transmitted-infections-say-doctors].

<u>4.5</u> Kitty Knowles, "Blaming dating apps for soaring STIs is a Luddite view," TheMemo.com, November 2, 2015 [last accessed on 9 July 2016 at http://www.thememo.com/2015/11/02/doctors-dating-apps-rise-in-sti-syphilis-gonorrhoea-sex/].

<u>4.6</u> Victoria Ward, "Dating apps 'to blame for rise in STIs and potential new HIV explosion' expert warns," *The Telegraph*, November 2, 2015 [last accessed on 9 July 2016 at http://www.telegraph.co.uk/news/health/11969699/Dating-apps-to-blame-for-rise-in-STIs-and-potential-new-HIV-explosion-expert-warns.html].

<u>4.7</u> AIDS Healthcare Foundation, "New AHF Billboard Campaign

Addresses STD Risks from Popular Dating Apps," September 24, 2015 [last accessed on 13 June 2016 at http://www.businesswire.com/news/home/20150924006283/en/AHF-Billboard-Campaign-Addresses-STD-Risks-Popular].

4.8 Stan Ziv, "Tinder Clashes with AIDS Healthcare Foundation over STD Billboard," *Newsweek*, September 30, 2015 [last accessed on 13 June 2016 at http://www.newsweek.com/tinder-clashes-aids-healthcare-foundation-over-std-billboard-378384]. To be fair to Tinder, AHF clearly has a fondness for latching onto to socially prominent brands to help spread its message; a current public service campaign uses the phrase "Feel the Burn?", which plays off the popular slogan for Democratic presidential candidate Bernie Sanders ("Feel the Bern").

4.9 AIDS Healthcare Foundation, "New AHF Billboard Campaign Addresses STD Risks from Popular Dating Apps," September 24, 2015 [last accessed on 13 June 2016 at http://www.businesswire.com/news/home/20150924006283/en/AHF-Billboard-Campaign-Addresses-STD-Risks-Popular]. Many if not most millennials are too young to remember bathhouses and the role that they played in the spread of HIV in the mid-1980s. Perhaps the most thorough and powerful examination of bathhouse culture and its role in the AIDS epidemic was written by Randy Shilts in his award-winning book, *And the Band Played On* (St. Martin's Press, 1987).

4.10 Ellen Brait, "Tinder and Grindr outraged over STD testing billboards that reference apps," *The Guardian*, September 29, 2015 [last accessed on 13 June 2016 at https://www.theguardian.com/technology/2015/sep/29/tinder-grindr-std-testing-aids-healthcare-foundation-billboards].

4.11 Letter from Jonathan D. Reichman to Michael Weinstein, September 18, 2015 [last accessed on 13 June 2016 at http://www.aidshealth.org/wp-content/uploads/2015/09/Ltr-re-False-Accusations-Against-Tinder-Inc..pdf].

4.12 Ellen Brait, "Tinder and Grindr outraged over STD testing billboards that reference apps," *The Guardian*, September 29, 2015 [last accessed on 13 June 2016 at https://www.theguardian.com/technology/2015/sep/29/tinder-grindr-std-testing-aids-healthcare-foundation-billboards].

4.13 Jose R. Gonzalez, "Dating App Tinder Adds STD Testing Locator After Pressure From AIDS Group," CNSNews.com, January 28, 2016 [last accessed on 13 June 2016 at http://www.cnsnews.com/news/article/jose-r-gonzalez/aids-foundation-pressures-dating-app-tinder-add-std-testing-locator-0]. Interestingly, the change did not merit a mention on the Tinder blog itself.

4.14 AIDS Healthcare Foundation, "AHF Applauds Tinder's Decision to Add Health Safety Section Including Healthvana's STD Testing Locator," January 21, 2016 [last accessed on 13 June 2016 at http://www.businesswire.com/news/home/20160121005939/en/AHF-Applauds-Tinder%E2%80%99s-Decision-Add-Health-Safety].

4.15 Ramin Bastani, email interview with the author, July 12, 2016.

4.16 Michael Smith, "Social Media and Disease: There's an App for That," The Gupta Guide, February 4, 2014 [last accessed on 2 July 2016 at http://www.medpagetoday.com/infectiousdisease/generalinfectiousdisease/].

4.17 "Tracking flu trends," Google Official Blog, November 11, 2008 [last accessed on 2 July 2016 at https://googleblog.blogspot.co.il/2008/11/tracking-flu-trends.html. Google announced on August 20, 2015 that it was shutting down the public version of Google Flu Trends and would devote itself to partnering with health organizations. "The Next Chapter for Flu Trends," Google Research Blog, August 20, 2015 [last accessed on 2 July 2016 at https://research.googleblog.com/2015/08/the-next-chapter-for-flu-trends.html].

4.18 "fertility," Def. 1, Merriam-Webster.com, [n.d.] [last accessed on 15 June 2016 at http://www.merriam-webster.com/dictionary/fertility].

4.19 "conception," Def. (a)1, Merriam-Webster.com, [n.d.] [last accessed on 15 June 2016 at http://www.merriam-webster.com/dictionary/conception].

4.20 "Pregnancy guide," WebMD, [n.d.] [last accessed on 16 June 2016 at http://www.webmd.boots.com/pregnancy/guide/getting-started-on-getting-pregnant].

4.21 Carolyn Kylstra, "22 Things You Should Know About STDs And Your Fertility" *BuzzFeed*, April 27, 2015 [last accessed on 16 June 2016 at https://www.buzzfeed.com/carolynkylstra/stds-and-infertility].

4.22 "How Sexually Transmitted Infections Affect Sperm Health," MyVMC, [n.d.] [last accessed on 16 June 2016 at http://www.myvmc.com/pregnancy/how-sexually-transmitted-infections-affect-sperm-health/].

4.23 Carolyn Kylstra, "22 Things You Should Know About STDs And

Your Fertility" *BuzzFeed*, April 27, 2015 [last accessed on 16 June 2016 at https://www.buzzfeed.com/carolynkylstra/stds-and-infertility].

4.24 "STDS AND INFERTILITY: PART 2", AttainFertility, [n.d.] [last accessed on 16 June 2016 at http://attainfertility.com/article/std-infertility-part-two].

4.25 *Id.*

4.26 "STDs during Pregnancy - CDC Fact Sheet" Centers for Disease Control, [n.d.] [last accessed on 17 June 2016 at http://www.cdc.gov/std/pregnancy/stdfact-pregnancy.htm].

4.27 Hallie Levine Sklar, "Pregnancy and STDs," *Parents*, April 2008 [last accessed on 3 July 2016 at http://www.parents.com/pregnancy/complications/infections/pregnancy-and-stds/].

4.28 "How to Prevent Sexually Transmitted Infections (STIs)," The American College of Obstetricians and Gynecologists, December 2015 [last accessed on 3 July 2016 at http://www.acog.org/~/media/For%20Patients/faq009.pdf; "How do sexually transmitted diseases and sexually transmitted infections (STDs/STIs) affect pregnancy?" Eunice Kennedy Shriver National Institute of Child Health and Human Development, May 28, 2013 [last accessed on 3 July 2016 at https://www.nichd.nih.gov/health/topics/stds/conditioninfo/Pages/infant.asp].

4.29 "STDs during Pregnancy - CDC Fact Sheet" Centers for Disease Control, [n.d.] [last accessed on 17 June 2016 at http://www.cdc.gov/std/pregnancy/stdfact-pregnancy.htm].

Endnotes for Chapter Five

5.1 "Birth and Natality," Centers for Disease Control and Prevention, February 25, 2016 [last accessed on 1 July 2016 at http://www.cdc.gov/nchs/fastats/births.htm. Births exceeded deaths in 2014 by nearly 1.5 million.

5.2 Ian Kerner, "Your smartphone may be powering down your relationship," CNN, January 10, 2013 [last accessed on 16 July 2016 at http://edition.cnn.com/2013/01/10/health/kerner-social-relationship/].

5.3 Barb Darrow, "Yes, your smartphone is hurting your love life:

study," *Fortune*, September 30, 2015 [last accessed on 16 July 2016 at http://fortune.com/2015/09/30/smartphones-hurt-your-love-life/].

5.4 Mandy Oaklander, "How Your Smartphone Is Ruining Your Relationship," *Time*, April 28, 2016 [last accessed on 16 July 2016 at http://time.com/4311202/smartphone-relationship-cell-phone/].

5.5 Mike Flacy, "ONE-THIRD OF AMERICANS PREFER THEIR SMARTPHONE OVER SEX," Digital Trends, August 3, 2011 [last accessed on 16 July 2016 at http://www.digitaltrends.com/android/one-third-of-americans-prefer-their-smartphone-over-sex/].

5.6 Haroon Siddique, "Britons having sex less often," *The Guardian*, November 26, 2013 [last accessed on 16 July 2013 at https://www.theguardian.com/society/2013/nov/26/britons-having-less-sex-recession-link-survey].

5.7 "Millennials spend one day every week on their phones - how can brands deal with the digital divide?" The Business Journals, November 19, 2015 [last accessed at http://www.bizjournals.com/prnewswire/press_releases/2015/11/19/C7321].

5.8 Michael Blaustein, "New study finds that 62% of women 'check phones during sex,'" *New York Post*, July 24, 2013 [last accessed on 16 July 2016 at http://nypost.com/2013/07/24/new-study-finds-that-62-of-women-check-phones-during-sex/].

5.9 Peter Wade, "Only 1 in 10 People Admit to Checking Their Phone During Sex," *Esquire*, May 14, 2016 [last accessed on 16 July 2016 at http://www.esquire.com/lifestyle/news/a44884/people-checking-their-phone-during-sex/].

5.10 Hallie Jackson, "Sleepless in America: How Digital Devices Keep Us Up All Night," NBC News, June 24, 2015 [last accessed on 16 July 2016 at http://www.nbcnews.com/nightly-news/sleepless-america-how-digital-devices-keep-us-all-night-n381251].

5.11 "Electronics in the Bedroom: Why it's Necessary to Turn off Before You Tuck in," National Sleep Foundation, [n.d.] [last accessed on 16 July 2016 at https://sleepfoundation.org/ask-the-expert/electronics-the-bedroom].

5.12 Taryn Hillin, "Here are all the ways sleep deprivation is killing your sex life," Fusion, March 18, 2015 [last accessed on 16 July 2016 at http://fusion.net/story/105433/here-are-all-the-ways-sleep-deprivation-is-killing-your-sex-life/].

5.13 Skye Gould and Kevin Loria, "Here's why the iPhone's Night Shift mode is such a big deal," Tech Insider, April 6, 2016 [last accessed on 16 July 2016 at http://www.techinsider.io/iphone-night-shift-blue-light-affects-your-brain-and-body-2016-4].

5.14 Chris Pleasance, "Don't sleep with your phone! NYPD tweets pics of charred pillows to warn about dangers of charging your cell in bed," *Daily Mail*, February 18, 2016 [last accessed on 4 July 2016 at http://www.dailymail.co.uk/news/article-3453519/Don-t-sleep-phone-NYPD-tweets-pics-charred-pillows-warn-dangers-charging-cell-bed.html].

5.15 *Id.*

5.16 princess-heya, "Hitachi magic wand caught on fire!," Reddit.com:TwoXChromosomes, April 11, 2014 [last accessed on 3 July 2016 at https://www.reddit.com/r/TwoXChromosomes/comments/22tbff/hitachi_m].

5.17 Sahara Rayne, "Could a vibrator get hot or explode?" AfraidtoAsk.com, August 18, 2015 [last accessed on 3 July 2016 at http://forums.afraidtoask.com/topic/29052/could-a-vibrator-get-hot-or-explode].

5.18 Gina Shaw, "Risky Business: Dangers of Sex Toys," Berkeley Wellness, June 25, 2015 [last accessed on 17 July 2016 at http://www.berkeleywellness.com/self-care/sexual-health/article/risky-business-dangers-sex-toys].

5.19 Liz Klinger, "Lioness Vibrator: Improve Your Sexual Experiences," Indiegogo, [n.d.] [last accessed on 2 July at https://www.indiegogo.com/projects/lioness-vibrator-improve-your-sexual-experiences--2#/].

5.20 "Jump Egg Sex Toy," Shenzhen Huifengsheng Technology Co., Ltd., [n.d.] [last accessed on 3 July 2016 at http://fengshenghui.en.alibaba.com/product/60406204199-801276518/Jump_Egg_Sex_Toys_Bluetooth_Wireless_App_Remote_Con].

5.21 Jonathan Plotzger, email to author, July 21, 2016.

5.22 Ellie Zolfagharifard, "Hackers could soon target SEX TOYS: Experts demonstrate how devices can be remotely controlled and even record video," *Daily Mail,* March 15, 2016 [last accessed on 18 July 2016 at http://www.dailymail.co.uk/sciencetech/article-3493426/How-hack-sex-toy-tech-firms-warn-public-growing-cyber-risks.html].

5.23 Sara Morrison, "'Smart' Dildo Company Sued For Tracking Users' Habits," vocativ, September 13, 2016 [last accessed on 21 September 2016 at http://www.vocativ.com/358530/smart-dildo-company-sued-for-tracking-users-habits/].

5.24 Nancy Jo Sales, "Tinder and the Dawn of the 'Dating Apocalypse,'" *Vanity Fair*, September 2015 [last accessed on 11 June 2016 at http://www.vanityfair.com/culture/2015/08/tinder-hook-up-culture-end-of-dating].

5.25 Emily Blatchford, "How Internet Porn Is Making Young Men Impotent," Huffington Post Australia, March 6, 2016 [last accessed on http://www.huffingtonpost.com.au/2016/06/02/how-internet-porn-is-making-young-men-impotent/].

5.26 Paolo Capogrosso MD, Michele Colicchia MD, Eugenio Ventimiglia MD, Giulia Castagna MD, Maria Chiara Clementi MD, Nazareno Suardi MD, Fabio Castiglione MD, Alberto Briganti MD, Francesco Cantiello MD, Rocco Damiano MD, Francesco Montorsi MD, andAndrea Salonia MD, "One Patient Out of Four with Newly Diagnosed Erectile Dysfunction Is a Young Man—Worrisome Picture from the Everyday Clinical Practice," *The Journal of Sexual Medicine*, July 2013 [last accessed on 5 July 2016 at http://onlinelibrary.wiley.com/doi/10.1111/jsm.12179/abstract].

5.27 Nicole Prause and James G. Pfaus, "Viewing Sexual Stimuli Associated with Greater Sexual Responsiveness, Not Erectile Dysfunction," *Sexual Medicine*, March 14, 2015 [last accessed on 5 July 2016 at https://www.researchgate.net/publication/269763975_Viewing_Sexual_Sti].

5.28 Monte Morin, "Study finds no link between viewing porn and erectile dysfunction," *Los Angeles Times*, March 17, 2016 [last accessed at http://www.latimes.com/science/sciencenow/la-sci-sn-porn-erection-20150316-story.html].

5.29 Daniel Engber, "Hands or Paws or Anything They Got," Slate.com, July 16, 2009 [last accessed on 5 July 2016 at http://www.slate.com/articles/health_and_science/science/2009/07/hands_c].

5.30 Mona Chalabi, "Dear Mona, I Masturbate More Than Once a Day. Am I Normal?" FiveThirtyEight, May 30, 2014 [last accessed on 5

July 2016 at http://fivethirtyeight.com/datalab/dear-mona-i-masturbate-more-than-once-a-day-am-i-normal/].

5.31 *Id.* Chalabi cited a self-study conducted by one young man who recorded the time spent on each masturbation session for a year. He concluded that he spent an average of almost 45 minutes each time he masturbated, or about 3% of his waking moments over the course of the year.

5.32 S.C. Boies, "University students' uses of and reactions to online sexual information and entertainment: Links to online and offline sexual behavior," *The Canadian Journal of Human Sexuality*, December 2001 [last accessed on 5 July 2016 at https://www.researchgate.net/publication/280055284_University_students'].

5.33 Ian Drury, "Alarm over teenage boys who have been warped by web porn: More than half of 11 to 16 year olds believe graphic images give a 'realistic' depiction of sex," *Daily Mail*, June 14, 2016 [last accessed on 19 July 2016 at http://www.dailymail.co.uk/news/article-3641879/Alarm-teenage-boys-warped-web-porn-half-11-16-year-olds-believe-graphic-images-realistic-depiction-sex.html].

5.34 Gail Dines, "Is porn immoral? That doesn't matter: It's a public health crisis," *Washington Post*, April 8, 2016 [last accessed on 19 July 2016 at https://www.washingtonpost.com/posteverything/wp/2016/04/08/is-porn-immoral-that-doesnt-matter-its-a-public-health-crisis/].

5.35 Justin Lehmiller, "Does Pornography Cause Men To Hate Women?" *Playboy,* September 9, 2015 [last accessed on 19 July 2016 at http://www.playboy.com/articles/adult-videos-men-hate-women].

Endnotes for Chapter Six

6.1 James M. Ambury, "Socrates (469—399 B.C.E.)," Internet Encyclopaedia of Philosophy, [n.d.] [last accessed on 7 July 2016 at http://www.iep.utm.edu/socrates/].

6.2 Juvenal, *Satires* (Satire VI, lines 347–8).

6.3 YoungPTone, "HR reading consistently high last few days," reddit.com/r/fitbit, February 4, 2016 [last accessed on 7 July 2016 at https://np.reddit.com/r/fitbit/comments/445ppj/hr_reading_consistently_hig

].

6.4 "Husband: Fitness band and Reddit revealed wife's pregnancy," BBC Radio 5 Live In Short, February 10, 2016 [last accessed on 7 July 2016 at http://www.bbc.co.uk/programmes/p03j4q40].

6.5 Alasdair Wilkins, "Do women avoid talking to their fathers because of evolution?" io9.com, November 29, 2010 [last accessed at http://io9.gizmodo.com/5701750/do-women-avoid-talking-to-their-fathers-because-of-evolution].

6.6 Colin Fernandez, "Fitness gadgets 'can track fertility': Devices could give women a 24-hour warning of the best time to try for a baby," *Daily Mail*, July 6, 2016 [last accessed on 7 July 2016 at http://www.dailymail.co.uk/health/article-3677718/Fitness-gadgets-track-fertility-Devices-women-24-hour-warning-best-time-try-baby-heart-rate-increases-ovulation.html].

6.7 Moira Wegel, "'Fitbit for Your Period': the rise of fertility tracking," *The Guardian*, March 23, 2016 [last accessed on 7 July 2016 at https://www.theguardian.com/technology/2016/mar/23/fitbit-for-your-period-the-rise-of-fertility-tracking].

6. "Signs and Symptoms of Ovulation," American Pregnancy Association, [n.d.] [last accessed on 8 July 2016 at http://americanpregnancy.org/getting-pregnant/signs-of-ovulation/].

6.9 Melissa Willets, "The 10 Best Fertility Apps," fitPregnancy.com, March 30, 2016 [last accessed on 8 July 2016 at http://www.fitpregnancy.com/pregnancy/getting-pregnant/best-fertility-apps].

6.10 "The HIPAA Privacy Rule," U.S. Department of Health and Human Services, [n.d.] [last accessed on 8 July 2016 at http://www.hhs.gov/hipaa/for-professionals/privacy/].

6.11 "MAKING SURE COMPANIES KEEP THEIR PRIVACY PROMISES TO CONSUMERS," Federal Trade Commission, [n.d.] [last accessed on 8 July 2016 at https://www.ftc.gov/news-events/media-resources/protecting-consumer-privacy/enforcing-privacy-promises].

6.12 Christine Magee, "VCs Find Fertile Ground In Women's Health," TechCrunch, July 15, 2014 [last accessed on 9 July 2016 at https://techcrunch.com/2014/07/15/vcs-find-fertile-ground-in-womens-health/].

Endnotes for Chapter Seven

7.1 "Creating Your Birth Plan," American Pregnancy Association, August 2015 [last accessed on 10 July 2016 at http://americanpregnancy.org/labor-and-birth/birth-plan/].

7.2 Stephanie Webber, "Kim Kardashian Documents Pregnancy Scare on Snapchat: 'Panic Attack,'" *US Weekly*, May 20, 2016 [last accessed on 10 July 2016 at http://www.usmagazine.com/celebrity-news/news/kim-kardashian-documents-pregnancy-scare-panic-attack-w207182].

7.3 "KIM KARDASHIAN Peed on Pregnancy Stick FOR FREE!" TMZ.com, May 20, 2016 [last accessed on 10 July 2016 at http://www.tmz.com/2016/05/20/kim-kardashian-clearblue-pregnancy-test/].

7.4 Kate Dries, "ClearBlue Is Now Paying Celebs to Tweet Their Pregnancy Tests," Jezebel, October 31, 2013 [last accessed on 10 July 2016 at http://jezebel.com/clearblue-is-now-paying-celebs-to-tweet-their-pregnancy-1456317435; Elise Solé, "Did These Celebs Really Sponsor Their Pregnancy Announcement?" Yahoo! Beauty, June 17, 2016 [last accessed on 10 July 2016 at https://www.yahoo.com/beauty/did-these-celebs-really-sponsor-1452941332308022.html].

7.5 Marisa Meltzer, "WombTube," Slate, March 14, 2011 [last accessed on 10 July 2016 at http://www.slate.com/articles/double_x/doublex/2011/03/wombtube.html].

7.6 Valerie Williams, "Posting A Positive Pregnancy Test On Social Media Is Gross, #SorryNotSorry," Mommyish.com, January 5, 2015 [last accessed on 10 July 2016 at http://www.mommyish.com/2015/01/05/dont-post-a-positive-pregnancy-test-on-facebook/].

7.7 Elizabeth Eden, "Pregnancy Tests Overview," HowStuffWorks Health, November 13, 2006 [last accessed on 10 July 2016 at http://health.howstuffworks.com/pregnancy-and-parenting/pregnancy/conception/how-pregnancy-tests-work.htm].

7.8 Alicia Barney, "Women Are Photoshopping Their Pregnancy Tests To Get Early Results," BuzzFeed, July 6, 2015 [last accessed on 10 July 2016 at https://www.buzzfeed.com/abarney/pregnancy-test-tweaking].

7.9 "Miscarriage," American Pregnancy Association, May 19, 2016 [last accessed on 10 July 2016 at http://americanpregnancy.org/pregnancy-complications/miscarriage/]; Dr. Susan Trout, "Chemical Pregnancy,"

PregnancyCorner.com, April 2016 [last accessed on 10 July 2016 at http://www.pregnancycorner.com/loss/chemical-pregnancy.html].

7.10 Buranda, "Announcing pregnancy on Facebook?" Mumsnet.com, March 1, 2011 [last accessed on 14 July 2016 at http://www.mumsnet.com/Talk/pregnancy/1161709-Announcing-pregnancy-on-Facebook].

7.11 "Miscarriage: Signs, causes, and treatment," BabyCenter.com, May 2015 [last accessed on 14 July 2016 at http://www.babycenter.com/0_miscarriage-signs-causes-and-treatment_252.bc].

7.12 brizzagirl, reply to "Announcing pregnancy on Facebook?" Mumsnet.com, March 1, 2011 [last accessed on 14 July 2016 at http://www.mumsnet.com/Talk/pregnancy/1161709-Announcing-pregnancy-on-Facebook].

7.13 George Gao and Gretchen Livingston, "Working while pregnant is much more common than it used to be," Pew Research Center, March 31, 2015 [last accessed on 14 July 2016 at http://www.pewresearch.org/fact-tank/2015/03/31/working-while-pregnant-is-much-more-common-than-it-used-to-be/].

7.14 Liz Morris, Cynthia Thomas Calvert, and Joan C. Williams, "What Young vs. UPS Means for Pregnant Workers and Their Bosses," *Harvard Business Review*, March 26, 2015 [last accessed on 14 July 2016 at https://hbr.org/2015/03/what-young-vs-ups-means-for-pregnant-workers-and-their-bosses].

Endnotes for Chapter Eight

8.1 North F, Ward WJ, Varkey P, Tulledge-Scheitel SM, "Should you search the Internet for information about your acute symptom?" *Telemedicine Journal and E-Health*, April 2012 [last accessed on 13 July 2016 at http://www.ncbi.nlm.nih.gov/pubmed/22364307].

8.2 Austin Frakt, "Using the Web or an App Instead of Seeing a Doctor? Caution Is Advised," *New York Times*, July 11, 2016 [last accessed on 13 July 2016 at http://www.nytimes.com/2016/07/12/upshot/using-the-web-or-an-app-before-seeing-a-doctor-caution-is-advised.html].

8.3 Steve Hoffenberg, "IBM's Watson Answers the Question, 'What's the Difference Between Artificial Intelligence and Cognitive Computing?'" VDCResearch.com, May 24, 2016 [last accessed on 13 July 2016 at http://www.vdcresearch.com/News-events/iot-blog/IBM-Watson-Answers-Question-Artificial-Intelligence.html].

    8.4 Michaeleen Doucleff, "Driving While Pregnant Is Riskier Than You Might Think," National Public Radio, May 12, 2014 [last accessed on 13 July 2016 at http://www.npr.org/sections/health-shots/2014/05/12/311862978/driving-while-pregnant-is-riskier-than-you-might-think].

    8.5 Nikhil Swarminathan, "Fact or Fiction?: Babies Exposed to Classical Music End Up Smarter," *Scientific American*, September 13, 2007 [last accessed on 13 July 2016 at http://www.scientificamerican.com/article/fact-or-fiction-babies-ex/].

    8.6 Denise Winterman, "Does Classical Music Make Babies Smarter?" BBC News Magazine, May 19, 2005 [last accessed on 13 July 2016 at http://news.bbc.co.uk/2/hi/4558507.stm].

    8.7 Nikhil Swarminathan, "Fact or Fiction?: Babies Exposed to Classical Music End Up Smarter," *Scientific American*, September 13, 2007 [last accessed on 13 July 2016 at http://www.scientificamerican.com/article/fact-or-fiction-babies-ex/].

    8.8 "'Mozart effect': can classical music really make your baby smarter?" *The Telegraph*, March 28, 2015 [last accessed on 13 July 2016 at http://www.telegraph.co.uk/news/health/children/11500314/Mozart-effect-can-classical-music-really-make-your-baby-smarter.html].

    8.9 Committee on Environmental Health, "Noise: A Hazard for Fetus and Newborn," *Pediatrics*, 1997 [last accessed on 13 July 2016 at http://pediatrics.aappublications.org/content/pediatrics/100/4/724.full.pdf].

    8.10 "Top 10 Noisiest Jobs," AccousticalSurfaces.com, [n.d.] [last accessed on 13 July 2016 at http://www.acousticalsurfaces.com/wp/assets/top-10-noisiest-jobs.jpg].

    https://consumer.healthday.com/health-technology-information-18/cellphone-health-news-729/does-mom-s-cellphone-startle-the-fetus-699055.html].

    8.12 *Id.*

    8.13 *Id.*

    8.14 Janny Scott, "Heat Exposure Increases the Chance of Birth Defects, Researchers Find," *Los Angeles Times,* May 3, 1991 [last accessed on 17 July 2016 at http://articles.latimes.com/1991-05-03/local/me-1121_1_tube-defect].

8.15 For a particularly clear explanation of this phenomenon, *see* hooj, reply to message by SemSevEr, "ELI5: Why do electronics (mainly computers) get hot when used extensively?" reddit.com, November 7, 2012 [last accessed on 17 July 2016 at https://www.reddit.com/r/explainlikeimfive/comments/12sgyk/eli5_why_d].

8.16 Matt Bach, "Gaming PC vs. Space Heater Efficiency," Puget Systems, October 21, 2013 [last accessed on 17 July 2016 at https://www.pugetsystems.com/labs/articles/Gaming-PC-vs-Space-Heater-Efficiency-511/].

8.17 Dr. Christopher S. Baird, "Why doesn't my laptop emit radiation?" Science Questions with Surprising Answers, December 4, 2014 [last accessed on 17 July 2016 at http://sciencequestionswithsurprisinganswers.org/2014/12/04/why-doesnt-my-laptop-emit-radiation/].

8.18 Bellieni CV, Pinto I, Bogi A, Zoppetti N, Andreuccetti D, Buonocore G., "Exposure to electromagnetic fields from laptop use of "laptop" computers," *Archives of Environmental & Occupational Health*, 2012 [last accessed on 17 July 2016 at http://www.ncbi.nlm.nih.gov/pubmed/22315933].

8.19 Sarah Wickline Wallan, "HypeWatch: Does Wi-Fi Really Disturb Fetal Brains?" MedPage Today, June 4, 2014 [last accessed on 17 July 2016 at http://www.medpagetoday.com/OBGYN/Pregnancy/46168].

8.20 David Coggan, "Wireless devices: a health threat during pregnancy?" *New Scientist*, June 9, 2014 [last accessed on 17 July 2016 at https://www.newscientist.com/article/dn25694-wireless-devices-a-health-threat-during-pregnancy/].

8.21 Darren Quick, "Study suggests mobile phone use during pregnancy may cause ADHD in offspring," Gizmag, March 19, 2012 [last accessed on 17 July 2016 at http://www.gizmag.com/mobile-phone-radiation-effects-fetus/21879/].

Endnotes for Chapter Nine

9.1 Siramaria, "The battle for privacy during pregnancy - a question of equality?" Reddit.com, May 27, 2015 [last accessed on 20 July 2015 at https://www.reddit.com/r/BabyBumps/comments/37gxr3/the_battle_for_pr].

9.2 pmf1985, in reply to Siramaria, "The battle for privacy during pregnancy - a question of equality?" Reddit.com, May 27, 2015 [last accessed on 20 July 2015 at https://www.reddit.com/r/BabyBumps/comments/37gxr3/the_battle_for_pr].

9.3 Charles Duhigg, "How Companies Learn Your Secrets," *New York Times Magazine*, February 16, 2016 [last accessed on 20 July 2016 at http://www.nytimes.com/2012/02/19/magazine/shopping-habits.html].

9.4 Sophie Curtis, "How much is your personal data worth?" *The Telegraph*, November 23, 2015 [last accessed on 20 July 2016 at http://www.telegraph.co.uk/technology/news/12012191/How-much-is-your-personal-data-worth.html].

9.5 Tim Chuey, "Everyone Complains About The Weather, But Nobody Does Anything About It," *Eugene Daily News,* April 4, 2016 [last accessed on 20 July 2016 at http://eugenedailynews.com/2016/04/everyone-complains-weather-nobody-anything/]. The history of this quote illustrates the peril of having a famous friend. The remark was initially made by Charles Dudley Warner, who co-authored *The Gilded Age: A Tale of Today* with his friend Mark Twain. Twain repeated the comment in a lecture and as a result, the quote is widely attributed to him.

9.6 Senator Jay Rockefeller (D-W.V.), "What Information Do Data Brokers Have on Consumers, and How Do They Use It?" Majority Statement, December 18, 2013 [last accessed on 20 July 2016 at http://www.commerce.senate.gov/public/index.cfm/hearings? ID=A5C3A62C-68A6-4735-9D18-916BDBBADF01].

9.7 Dan Goodin, "User data plundering by Android and iOS apps is as rampant as you suspected," ArsTechnica, November 4, 2015 [last accessed on 19 August 2016 at http://arstechnica.com/security/2015/11/user-data-plundering-by-android-and-ios-apps-is-as-rampant-as-you-suspected/].

9.8 Janet Vertesi, "My Experiment Opting Out of Big Data Made Me Look Like a Criminal," *Time*, May 1, 2014 [last accessed on 22 July 2016 at http://time.com/83200/privacy-internet-big-data-opt-out/].

9.9 Megan Treacy, "GPS becomes accurate down to a few centimeters," treehugger, February 15, 2016 [last accessed on 22 July

2016 at http://www.treehugger.com/gadgets/gps-becomes-accurate-down-centimeter.html].

9.10 Danielle Citron, "BEWARE: The Dangers Of Location Data," *Forbes*, December 24, 2014 [last accessed on 19 August 2016 at http://www.forbes.com/sites/daniellecitron/2014/12/24/beware-the-dangers-of-location-data/#7a6481a69685].

Endnotes for Chapter Ten

10.1 George Lois, "FLASHBACK: DEMI MOORE," *Vanity Fair*, August 2011 [last accessed on 24 July 2016 at http://www.vanityfair.com/news/2011/08/demi-moore-201108].

10.2 Rebecca Pocklington, "Scout Willis strips topless and walks through New York in protest against Instagram's anti-nudity rules, " *Mirror*, May 28, 2014 [last accessed on 24 July 2016 at http://www.mirror.co.uk/3am/celebrity-news/scout-willis-strips-topless-walks-3618884].

10.3 Nora Crotty, "A HISTORY OF NAKED, PREGNANT CELEBS ON MAGAZINE COVERS," Fashionista, March 7, 2012 [last accessed on 24 July 2016 at http://fashionista.com/2012/03/a-history-of-naked-pregnant-celebs-on-magazine-covers].

10.4 "deekaygee," March 1, 2015 comment in response to "Don't want to flaunt the bump …," WhatToExpect.com, [n.d.] [last accessed on 26 July 2016 at http://www.whattoexpect.com/forums/may-2015-babies/topic/don-39-t-want-to-flaunt-the-bump.html].

10.5 Patricia Garcia, "Stop Asking Me to Post Photos of My Baby Bump on Instagram," *Vogue*, November 4, 2014 [last accessed on 24 July 2016 at http://www.vogue.com/3622347/pregnancy-reveals-social-media/].

10.6 Chrissy Teigen, post on Instagram, October 18, 2015 [last accessed on 21 August 2016 at https://www.instagram.com/p/8_CUaFJjd1/].

10.7 Lindsay Kimble, "Chrissy Teigen Swears Off Tweeting About Pregnancy After Body-Shamers Attack Her Baby Bump," *People*, October 18, 2015 [last accessed on 22 August 2016 at http://celebritybabies.people.com/2015/10/18/chrissy-teigen-baby-bump-photo-replies-to-body-shamers/].

10.8 Brittany Aäe, post on Instagram, June 1, 2016 [last accessed on 22 August 2016 at https://www.instagram.com/p/BGF62BwJ5jx/].

10.9 Meg Ireland, email to author, June 21, 2016.

10.10 Daniel Piotrowski, "Pregnant mum disgusted to learn her photo was stolen by a Facebook creep and used to lure viewers to 'PREGGOPHILA' fetish site," *Daily Mail*, August 14, 2015 [last accessed on 22 August 2016 at http://www.dailymail.co.uk/news/article-3197504/Mother-shocked-picture-stolen-PREGGOPHILE-fetish-website.html].

10.11 Lisa Vaas, "Pregnancy groups warn of 'Preggophiles' stealing Facebook photos of baby bumps," Naked Security by Sophos, August 14, 2015 [last accessed on 23 August 2016 at https://nakedsecurity.sophos.com/2015/08/14/pregnancy-groups-warn-of-preggophiles-stealing-facebook-photos-of-baby-bumps/].

10.12 Meg Ireland, email to author, June 21, 2016.

10.13 "Mary," February 16, 2011 comment in response to Jenny Hwang, "Ultrasound Pictures on Facebook: Creepy and Inappropriate?" GeekInHeels.com, May 25, 2010 [last accessed on 26 July 2016 at http://www.geekinheels.com/2010/05/25/ultrasound-pictures-on-facebook-creepy-and-inappropriate.html/].

10.14 Madlen Davies, "The baby scan selfie craze: Rise in pregnant women posting pictures online inviting others to guess their unborn child's sex," *Daily Mail*, December 30, 2014 [last accessed on 26 July 2016 at http://www.dailymail.co.uk/health/article-2890284/Mothers-posting-scan-pictures-online-asking-guess-sex.html].

10.15 Email from Dr. Zhenya Pozharny to the author, August 20, 2016.

Endnotes for Chapter Eleven

11.1 Eric Limer, "The First Text Message Was Sent 20 Years Ago Today," Gizmodo, December 3, 2012 [last accessed on 20 September 2016 at http://gizmodo.com/5965121/the-first-text-message-was-sent-20-years-ago-today].

11.2 Helena Horton, "Man catches a Pidgey on Pokémon GO as his wife gives birth," *The Telegraph*, July 8, 2016 [last accessed on 19 July 2016 at http://www.telegraph.co.uk/technology/2016/07/08/man-catches-a-pidgey-on-pokmon-go-as-his-wife-gives-birth/]. The photo was posted to the Web site Imgur, where it has been viewed over a million times.

11.3 Maria Bailey, "#PokemonGoProblems: Players share their game obsession in hilarious photos," *NY Daily News*, July 13, 2016 [last accessed on 20 July 2016 at http://www.nydailynews.com/entertainment/pokemongoproblems-players-share-game-obsession-hilarious-photos-gallery-1.2709734?pmSlide=1.2709721].

11.4 Tina Cassidy, "Texting While Birthing," *New York Magazine*, February 4, 2011 [last accessed on 23 July 2016 at http://nymag.com/news/intelligencer/71283/].

11.5 Jeanne Sager, "Texting in the Delivery Room: Does Birth Really Need to Be Social?" The Stir, February 13, 2011 [last accessed on 23 July 2016 at http://thestir.cafemom.com/pregnancy/116097/texting_in_the_delivery_roo].

11.6 Laura Hudson, "Q&A: Claire Diaz-Ortiz, the Woman Who Got the Pope on Twitter," *Wired*, December 17, 2012 [last accessed on 23 July 2016 at http://www.wired.com/2012/12/pope-twitter-interview/].

11.7 Laura Stampler, "Twitter Employee Live Tweets Her Baby's Birth Because … Twitter," *Time*, April 7, 2014 [last accessed on 23 July 2016 at http://time.com/51689/twitter-employee-live-tweets-her-babys-birth-because-twitter/].

11.8 Ali Vingiano, "A Twitter Employee Live-Tweeted Giving Birth" BuzzFeed, April 5, 2014 [last accessed on 23 July 2016 at https://www.buzzfeed.com/alisonvingiano/twitter-employee-live-tweeting-labor].

11.9 Paul Bentley, "Mother-to-be who invited millions into the delivery room … via Twitter: Lyndsey shares pictures of herself posing with doctors, suffering contractions and having epidural during 12-hour labour," *Daily Mail*, June 8, 2014 [last accessed on 23 July 2016 at http://www.dailymail.co.uk/news/article-2652317/Mother-shares-pictures-posing-doctors-suffering-contractions-having-epidural-12-hour-labour-Twitter.html].

11.10 Doree Shafrir, "This Is The Most Amazing Home Birth Story You'll Ever Read," BuzzFeed, January 8, 2016 [last accessed at 23 July 2016 at https://www.buzzfeed.com/doree/this-san-francisco-man-delivered-his-wifes-baby-at-home].

11.11 Alyssa Newcomb, "First-Time Mom Live-Tweets Birth With Unflinching Honesty, Tweets Go Viral," ABC News, January 10, 2014 [last accessed on 23 July 2016 at http://abcnews.go.com/blogs/health/2014/01/10/first-time-mom-live-tweets-birth-with-unflinching-honesty-tweets-go-viral/].

11.12 Ruth Fowler, "How I Went From 'Poster Mother' to Pariah," The Daily Dose, August 17, 2015 [last accessed on 23 July 2016 at http://www.damemagazine.com/2015/08/17/how-i-went-poster-mother-pariah].

11.13 Kevin Maney, "Baby's arrival inspires birth of cellphone camera — and societal evolution," *USA Today*, January 23, 2007 [last accessed on 22 July 2016 at http://usatoday30.usatoday.com/tech/columnist/kevinmaney/2007-01-23-kahn-cellphone-camera_x.htm].

11.14 Katharine Q. Seelye, "Cameras, and Rules Against Them, Stir Passions in Delivery Rooms," *New York Times*, February 2, 2011 [last accessed on 23 July 2016 at http://www.nytimes.com/2011/02/03/us/03birth.html].

11.15 Alice Johnston, "He's brave! Man wears a T-shirt with 'I did this to you' WHILE his wife is in labour — and she does not look pleased," *Daily Mail*, June 27, 2016 [last accessed on 26 July 2016 at http://www.dailymail.co.uk/femail/article-3661992/He-s-brave-Man-wears-T-shirt-did-wife-labour-does-not-look-pleased.html].

11.16 Bianca London, "She already has one baby! Brave (and silly) man poses for a smiling SELFIE while his wife gives birth in the background," *Daily Mail*, November 10, 2015 [last accessed on 26 July 2016 at http://www.dailymail.co.uk/femail/article-3312001/Brave-man-poses-smiling-SELFIE-wife-gives-birth-background-viral-photo-sweeping-internet.html].

11.17 Tiare Dunlap, "Man Who Streamed Son's Birth on Facebook Live Didn't Know He Was Sharing It with the World: 'I Thought It Was Just Going to My Family,' *People*, May 18, 2016 [last accessed on 24 August 2016 at http://www.people.com/article/facebook-live-birth-dad-who-streamed-sons-entire-birth-didnt-know-he-shared-with-world].

11.18 Kirstie McCrum, "Dad-to-be who streamed child's birth on Facebook Live says he had no idea it was being broadcast," *Daily Mirror*, May 19, 2016 [last accessed on 20 September 2016 at http://www.mirror.co.uk/news/world-news/dad-who-streamed-childs-birth-8006457].

11.19 Jessica Remitz, "Birth Announcement Etiquette — Don't Mess This Up!" *Parents*, November 11, 2015 [last accessed on 22 July 2016 at http://www.parents.com/pregnancy/my-life/birth-announcements/birth-announcement-etiquette/].

Endnotes for Chapter Twelve

12.1 Bonnie Rochman, "Baby Name Game: How a Name Can Affect Your Child's Future," *Time*, December 2, 2011 [last accessed on 18 July 2016 at http://healthland.time.com/2011/12/02/how-baby-names-affect-your-childs-future/].

12.2 Pamela Redmond Satran And Linda Rosenkrantz, "How Important Is a Name?" Parenting, September 3, 2004 [last accessed on 18 July 2016 at http://www.parenting.com/article/how-important-is-a-name].

12.3 Doris Maria Bregolisse, "Website named baby born to Kelowna couple," Global News, April 10, 2014 [last accessed on 18 July 2016 at http://globalnews.ca/news/1263872/website-named-baby-born-to-kelowna-couple/].

12.4 digitalgecko, "IAmA Crazy man trying to let the internet name my daughter... Yes my wife knows," Reddit.com, January 11, 2014 [last accessed on 18 July 2016 at https://www.reddit.com/r/casualiama/comments/1uyzb9/iama_crazy_man_].

12.5 "Top 15 Most Popular Search Engines," eBiz, July 2016 [last accessed on 24 July 2016 at http://www.ebizmba.com/articles/search-engines].

12.6 Vinny La Barbera, "8 SEO Stats That Are Hard to Ignore," imFORZA, April 19, 2012 [last accessed on 24 July 2016 at https://www.imforza.com/blog/8-seo-stats-that-are-hard-to-ignore/].

12.7 Allen Salkin, "What's in a Name? Ask Google," *New York Times*, November 25, 2011 [last accessed on 24 July 2016 at http://www.nytimes.com/2011/11/27/fashion/google-searches-help-parents-narrow-down-baby-names.html].

12.8 Marlin Bressi, "5 Most Common Names Chosen By Adult Film Actresses," Wikinut, January 19, 2012 [last accessed on 11 September 2016 at http://humour.wikinut.com/5-Most-Common-Names-Chosen-By-

Adult-Film-Actresses/1egw.o2y/].

12.9 Like so many Yogiisms, this line predates Berra but he made it famous. Garson O'Toole, "Nobody Goes There Anymore, It's Too Crowded," Quote Investigator, August 29, 2014 [last accessed on 25 August 2016 at http://quoteinvestigator.com/2014/08/29/too-crowded/].

12.10 Benton Lane, email with author, August 6, 2016.

Endnotes for Chapter Thirteen

13.1 Jennifer Langston, "Family technology rules: What kids expect of parents," *UWToday*, March 8, 2016 [last accessed on 30 August 2016 at http://www.washington.edu/news/2016/03/08/family-technology-rules-what-kids-expect-of-parents/].

13.2 Julia Fierro, "That Time a Photo of My 2-Year-Old Daughter Went Viral," Huffington Post, June 2, 2014 [last accessed on 1 September 2016 at http://www.huffingtonpost.com/julia-fierro/a-photo-of-my-2-year-old-daughter-went-viral_b_5400506.html].

13.3 Christie Hoos, "My Child's Photo was Used in an Offensive Corporate Campaign," So Here's Us …, June 12, 2015 [last accessed on 1 September 2016 at https://soheresus.com/2015/06/12/down-syndrome-genoma-copyright-infringement/].

13.4 Blake Miller, "The Creepiest New Corner Of Instagram: Role-Playing With Stolen Baby Photos," *Fast Company*, September 23, 2014 [last accessed on 2 September 2016 at http://www.fastcompany.com/3036073/the-creepiest-new-corner-of-instagram-role-playing-with-stolen-baby-photos].

13.5 Nick Whigham, "Digital kidnapping will make you think twice about what you post to social media," news.com.au, July 21, 2015 [last accessed on 2 September 2016 at http://www.news.com.au/lifestyle/real-life/wtf/digital-kidnapping-will-make-you-think-twice-about-what-you-post-to-social-media/news-story/4dc1c9a22b657f090c25c9393f66fe88].

13.6 Blake Miller, "The Creepiest New Corner Of Instagram: Role-Playing With Stolen Baby Photos," *Fast Company*, September 23, 2014 [last accessed on 2 September 2016 at http://www.fastcompany.com/3036073/the-creepiest-new-corner-of-instagram-role-playing-with-stolen-baby-photos].

13.7 "Parents discover children's Facebook photos on Russian paedophile website," *The Telegraph*, January 13, 2015 [last accessed on 7 August 2016 at http://www.telegraph.co.uk/news/uknews/crime/11342175/Parents-discover-childrens-Facebook-photos-on-Russian-paedophile-website.html].

13.8 Harry Wallop, "Why the idea of paedophiles stealing pictures of my kids doesn't bother me," *The Telegraph*, January 15, 2015 [last accessed on 7 August 2016 at http://www.telegraph.co.uk/men/relationships/fatherhood/11345624/Why-the-idea-of-paedophiles-stealing-pictures-of-my-kids-doesnt-bother-me.html].

13.9 Sara Hall, January 15, 2015, comment in response to Harry Wallop, "Why the idea of paedophiles stealing pictures of my kids doesn't bother me," *The Telegraph*, January 15, 2015 [last accessed on 7 August 2016 at http://www.telegraph.co.uk/men/relationships/fatherhood/11345624/Why-the-idea-of-paedophiles-stealing-pictures-of-my-kids-doesnt-bother-me.html].

13.10 David Chazan, "French parents 'could be jailed' for posting children's photos online," *The Telegraph*, March 1, 2016 [last accessed on 5 August 2016 at http://www.telegraph.co.uk/news/worldnews/europe/france/12179584/Fren parents-could-be-jailed-for-posting-childrens-photos-online.html].

13.11 *Id.*

13.12 "Woman sues parents for sharing embarrassing childhood photos," The Local AT, September 14, 2016 [last accessed on 21 September 2016 at http://www.thelocal.at/20160914/woman-sues-parents-for-sharing-embarrassing-childhood-photos-on-facebook]. Since the story first ran, some questions have been raised about whether a suit has actually been filed: "Doubts cast over alleged Facebook court case," The Local AT, September 16, 2016 [last accessed on 21 September 2016 at http://www.thelocal.at/20160916/doubts-cast-over-alleged-facebook-court-case].

13.13 Matt Werman and David Barrett, "Google must delete your data if you ask, EU rules," *The Telegraph*, May 13, 2014 [last accessed on 5 August 2016 at http://www.telegraph.co.uk/technology/google/10827005/Google-must-delete-your-data-if-you-ask-EU-rules.html].

13.14 "iRights launch," UK Safer Internet Center, July 28, 2015 [last accessed on 5 August 2016 at http://www.saferinternet.org.uk/news/irights].

13.15 Cheryl Lock, "How to Protect Your Kid's Photos Online," *Parents*, June 11, 2015 [last accessed on 6 August 2016 at http://www.parents.com/fun/arts-crafts/photography/protect-kid-photos-online/].

Endnotes for Chapter Fourteen

14.1 David Priest, "Hatch Baby Smart Changing Pad review," c|net, May 14, 2016 [last accessed on 31 July 2016 at http://www.cnet.com/products/hatch-baby-smart-changing-pad/].

14.2 Gretchen McCord, "Choose Privacy Week 2015: What You Should Know About 'Anonymous' Aggregate Data About You," Choose Privacy Week, May 5, 2015 [last accessed on 31 July 2016 at https://chooseprivacyweek.org/choose-privacy-week-2015-what-you-should-know-about-anonymous-aggregate-data-about-you/].

14.3 Lauren Walker, "HELLO BARBIE, YOUR CHILD'S CHATTIEST AND RISKIEST CHRISTMAS PRESENT," *Newsweek*, December 15, 2015 [last accessed on 1 August 2016 at http://www.newsweek.com/2015/12/25/hello-barbie-your-childs-chattiest-and-riskiest-christmas-present-404897.html].

14.4 Wendy Morelli, "10 Best Baby Apps for New Parents, From Baby Monitors to Lullabies," iVillage.com, [n.d.] [last accessed on 4 September 2016 at http://www.ivillage.ca/parenting/stuff-we-love/10-best-baby-apps-new-parents-baby-monitors-lullabies].

14.5 Kashmir Hill, "'Baby Monitor Hack' Could Happen To 40,000 Other Foscam Users," *Forbes*, August 27, 2013 [last accessed on 27 July 2016 at http://www.forbes.com/sites/kashmirhill/2013/08/27/baby-monitor-hack-could-happen-to-40000-other-foscam-users/].

14.6 "Seen at 11: Cyber Spies Could Target Your Child Through a Baby Monitor," CBS New York, April 21, 2015 [last accessed on 27 July 2016 at http://newyork.cbslocal.com/2015/04/21/seen-at-11-cyber-spies-could-target-your-child-through-a-baby-monitor/].

14.7 Kayla Keegan, "Someone Hacked This Family's Baby Monitor—and Posted The Footage Online" *Redbook*, April 6, 2015 [last accessed on

27 July 2016 at http://www.redbookmag.com/life/friends-family/news/a21290/this-family-finds-out-that/].

14.8 Leo Kelion, "Breached webcam and baby monitor site flagged by watchdogs," BBC News, November 21, 2014 [last accessed on 27 July 2016 at http://www.bbc.com/news/technology-30121159].

Endnotes for Chapter Fifteen

15.1 David Priest, "4moms mamaRoo review," c|net, May 11, 2016 [last accessed on 1 August 2016 at http://www.cnet.com/products/4moms-mamaroo/].

15.2 "SIDS and Other Sleep-Related Infant Deaths: Expansion of Recommendations for a Safe Infant Sleeping Environment," American Academy of Pediatrics, October 17, 2011 [last accessed on 1 August 2016 at http://pediatrics.aappublications.org/content/pediatrics/early/2011/10/12/pe2284.full.pdf].

15.3 Clemence Michallon, "How far would YOU go to catch'em all? New York tech exec, 28, becomes the first person to catch all 145 Pokemon across the globe," *Daily Mail*, August 5, 2016 [last accessed on 7 August 2016 at http://www.dailymail.co.uk/news/article-3725461/How-far-catch-em-New-York-tech-exec-28-catch-Pokemon-United-States-takes-quest-Paris-Hong-Kong-Sydney.html].

15.4 "Toddler, 2, is found crying and wandering outside after parents leave him home alone for TWO hours while playing Pokemon Go," *Daily Mail*, August 1, 2016 [last accessed on 7 August 2016 at http://www.dailymail.co.uk/news/article-3718425/Toddler-2-crying-wandering-outside-parents-leave-home-TWO-hours-playing-Pokemon-Go.html].

15.5 Joe Nerssessian, "Parents' smartphone obsession putting children at risk, warns senior paediatrician," *Independent*, June 6, 2016 [last accessed on 29 July 2016 at http://www.independent.co.uk/life-style/gadgets-and-tech/parents-smartphone-obsession-putting-children-at-risk-warns-senior-paediatrician-a7066926.html].

15.6 Jesse Singal, "Are Cell-Phone-Distracted Parents Really Endangering Kids at the Playground?" *New York Magazine*, April 27, 2015 [last accessed on 29 July 2016 at http://nymag.com/scienceofus/2015/04/new-study-makes-all-parents-feel-guilty.html].

15.7 Varda Epstein, "Distracted Parenting — These Stats Will Get Your Attention," Kars4Kids.com, March 31, 2014 [last accessed on 29 July 2016 at http://www.kars4kids.org/blog/distracted-parenting-stats-will-get-attention/].

15.8 Elizabeth Aguilera, "Too much 'brexting' undermines bonding during breastfeeding," Southern California Public Radio, September 24, 2015 [last accessed on 15 August 2015 at http://www.scpr.org/news/2015/09/24/54595/brexting-impacts-baby-bonding-during-breastfeeding/].

15.9 Tanvier Peart, "Why Brexting (Breastfeeding & Texting) Is a Very Bad Idea," The Stir, September 25, 2015 [last accessed on 16 August 2016 at http://thestir.cafemom.com/baby/191034/brexting_moms_who_breastfeed].

15.10 Sophie Haslett, "Are YOU guilty of 'brexting'? Mothers shamed for using their smartphone while breastfeeding because it interferes with bonding," *Daily Mail*, May 2, 2016 [last accessed on 15 August 2016 at http://www.dailymail.co.uk/femail/article-3568929/Are-guilty-brexting-s-browsing-smartphone-breastfeed-countless-mothers-shamed-for.html].

15.11 Elizabeth Aguilera, "Too much 'brexting' undermines bonding during breastfeeding," Southern California Public Radio, September 24, 2015 [last accessed on 15 August 2015 at http://www.scpr.org/news/2015/09/24/54595/brexting-impacts-baby-bonding-during-breastfeeding/].

15.12 "IU study finds infant attention span suffers when parents' eyes wander during playtime," IU Bloomington Newsroom, April 28, 2016 [last accessed on 15 August 2016 at http://news.indiana.edu/releases/iu/2016/04/infant-attention-span.shtml].

Endnotes for Chapter Sixteen

16.1 laney_bee, "I dropped my iPhone on my baby!!!!!!" babycenter. community, December 17, 2011 [last accessed on 17 August 2016 at http://community.babycenter.com/post/a30754775/i_dropped_my_iphone_].

16.2 Bonnie Rochman, "Pediatricians Say Cell Phone Radiation Standards Need Another Look," *Time*, July 20, 2012 [last accessed on 16 August 2016 at http://healthland.time.com/2012/07/20/pediatricians-call-on-the-fcc-to-reconsider-cell-phone-radiation-standards/].

16.3 Robert J. Szczerba, "Controversial Paper Suggests Wi-Fi Exposure More Dangerous To Kids Than Previously Thought," *Forbes*, January 13, 2016 [last accessed on 16 August 2016 at http://www.forbes.com/sites/robertszczerba/2015/01/13/study-suggests-wi-fi-exposure-more-dangerous-to-kids-than-previously-thought/].

16.4 Lloyd Morgan, Santosh Kesari, and Devra Lee Davis, "Why children absorb more microwave radiation than adults: The consequences," *Journal of Microscopy and Ultrastructure*, December 2014 [last accessed on 16 August 2015 at http://www.sciencedirect.com/science/article/pii/S2213879X14000583].

16.5 Ian Douglas, "Wi-Fi is not harming our chidren - here's the evidence," *The Telegraph*, May 13, 2015 [last accessed on 17 August 2016 at http://www.telegraph.co.uk/women/mother-tongue/11599311/Wi-Fi-is-not-harming-our-chidren-heres-the-evidence.html].

16.6 Thomas Tamblyn, "Study Claims WiFi Is 'More Dangerous' To Kids," Huffpost Tech UK, January 14, 2015 [last accessed on 17 August 2016 at http://www.huffingtonpost.co.uk/2015/01/14/study-wifi-dangerous-to-children_n_6468586.html].

16.7 Akemi Iwaya, "Could Wi-Fi be Harmful to a Newborn Baby?" How-To Geek, February 20, 2014 [last accessed on 17 August 2016 at http://www.howtogeek.com/183031/could-wi-fi-be-harmful-to-a-newborn-baby/].

16.8 Daniela Ongaro, "Your child's phone and tablet could be harming their eyes, expert warns,' *The Daily Telegraph*, August 24, 2014 [last accessed on 17 August 2016 at http://www.dailytelegraph.com.au/entertainment/arts/your-childs-phone-and-tablet-could-be-harming-their-eyes-expert-warns/news-story/c91174a8dcd55d0e70f0836144a403c5].

16.9 Ciaran Haughton, Mary Aiken, and Carly Cheevers, "Cyber Babies: The Impact of Emerging Technology on the Developing Infant," *Psychology Research*, September 2015 [last accessed on 13 September 2016 at http://www.davidpublisher.com/Public/uploads/Contribute/5643e8fa5b797].

16.10 Jeanie Lerche Davis, "Computers Hurt Kids' Eyes," WebMD, March 26, 2002 [last accessed on 17 August 2016 at http://www.webmd.com/baby/news/20020326/computers-hurt-kids-eyes].

16.11 Heidi Evans, "Toddlers may be at risk from technology, warn experts as new study shows use soars by diaper set," *New York Daily News*, April 7, 2014 [last accessed on 14 September 2016 at http://www.nydailynews.com/news/national/toddlers-risk-tech-experts-study-shows-soars-article-1.1747694].

16.12 Maggie Fox, "Toddlers Are Already Pros With Tablets And Smartphones, Study Finds," NBC News, November 3, 2015 [last accessed on 14 September 2016 at http://www.nbcnews.com/health/kids-health/toddlers-are-already-pros-tablets-smartphones-study-finds-n455881].

16.13 Luke Dormehl, "Psychologist: Giving your kid an iPad is 'child abuse,'" Cult of Mac, September 23, 2015 [last accessed on 14 September 2016 at http://www.cultofmac.com/389895/psychologist-giving-your-kid-an-ipad-is-child-abuse/].

16.14 James Covert, "Holiday Monster," *New York Post*, December 24, 2012 [last accessed on 15 September 2016 at http://nypost.com/2012/12/24/holiday-monster/].

16.15 "Why Are Physical Educational Toys Better for Young Children," Spielgaben, July 20, 2015 [last accessed on 15 September 2016 at https://spielgaben.com/why-are-physical-educational-toys-better-for-young-children/].

16.16 "Imagination important for children's cognitive development," *Harvard Gazette*, March 1, 2002 [last accessed on 15 September 2016 at http://news.harvard.edu/gazette/story/2002/03/imagination-important-for-childrens-cognitive-development/].

16.17 Scott Barry Kaufman Ph.D., "The Need for Pretend Play in Child Development," *Psychology Today,* March 6, 2012 [last accessed on 15 September 2016 at https://www.psychologytoday.com/blog/beautiful-minds/201203/the-need-pretend-play-in-child-development].

16.18 Bertrand Russell, *Education and the Good Life* (New York: Avon Book Division, 1926), p. 21.

16.19 George Bernard Shaw, *Back to Methuselah*, act I, from *Selected Plays with Prefaces*, vol. 2, p. 7 (1949).

16.20 "empathy," *Merriam-Webster Learner's Dictionary*, 2016 [last accessed on 12 August 2016 at http://www.merriam-webster.com/dictionary/empathy].

16.21 Walter McKenzie, "Empathy: the most important 21st Century Skill," ASCD Edge, June 20, 2011 [last accessed on 16 September 2016 at http://edge.ascd.org/blogpost/empathy-the-most-important-21st-century-skill].

16.22 Claire Lerner and Rebecca Parlakian, "How to Help Your Child Develop Empathy," Zero to Three, February 1, 2016 [last accessed on 16 September 2016 at https://www.zerotothree.org/resources/5-how-to-help-your-child-develop-empathy].

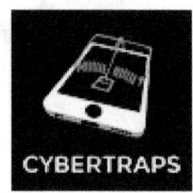

Disclaimer

This e-book **DOES NOT** constitute legal advice, nor does it express a legal opinion about any particular set of facts. Your purchase of this e-book does not create an attorney-client relationship with the author. If you are facing any of the situations described in this e-book, or think that any of the legal principles discussed might apply to your particular circumstances, you are STRONGLY URGED to seek professional counsel from an attorney licensed to practice law in the jurisdiction in which you reside, and in particular, to get counsel from an attorney experienced in the practice of educational law.

As the author of this e-book, I have made reasonable efforts to include accurate information regarding legislation, cases, and other legal developments; nonetheless, errors or omissions may occur. Moreover, as the law in the United States varies from state to state, and from state jurisdictions to the federal government, a correct statement of the law in one jurisdiction may not be accurate as to other jurisdictions.

To the best of my ability, the material contained in this e-book is accurate as of the date of publication. However, the law continually changes, as new legislation is passed and new decisions are handed down by the courts. You are advised that despite my best efforts, the information contained in this e-book may be out of date. I have no legal obligation to revise or update this e-book, although I may choose to do so. In the event that this e-book is updated, subsequent editions will be so identified.

The purpose of this e-book is to provide general information on the topics herein and to communicate my personal opinions and experience with respect to fascinating issues raised by the emergence of new technologies in our society.

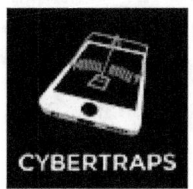

CYBERTRAPS

About the Author

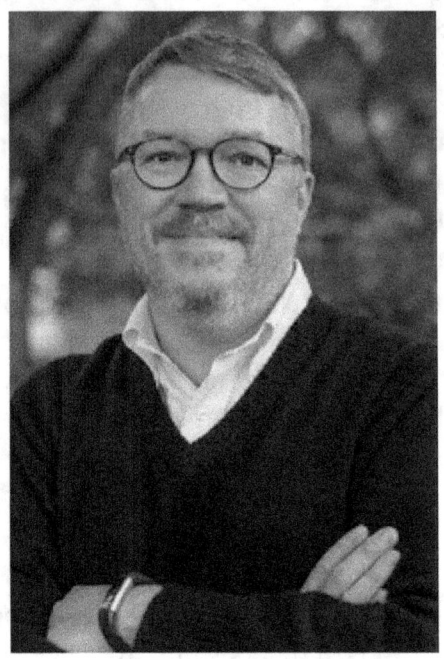

I am an author, attorney, expert witness, and professional speaker on the legal and cultural implications of emerging technology, with a particular focus on law, privacy, cybersafety, and ethics. After graduating from Amherst College and Boston College Law School, I clerked for two years for the Honorable Frank H. Freedman, Chief Judge of the U.S. District Court in Massachusetts. After practicing law for five years and writing my first book, *Vermont Jury Instructions — Civil and Criminal* [with John Dinse and Ritchie Berger] (Butterworths 1993), I launched a computer consulting business that in turn led to my current work as an author, lecturer, and computer forensics expert.

In response to the passage of the Communications Decency Act in 1996, I began researching the legislative and media response to the rise of the online adult industry. The resulting book, *Obscene Profits: The Entrepreneurs of Pornography in the Cyber Age* (Routledge 2000), was the first of what are now six mainstream non-fiction books. The others are:

- *The Naked Employee: How Technology Is Compromising Workplace Privacy* (Amacom 2003);
- *The Decency Wars: The Campaign to Cleanse American Culture* (Prometheus Books 2006);
- *The Court and the Cross: The Religious Right's Crusade to Reshape the Supreme Court* (Beacon Press 2008);
- *American Privacy: The 400-Year History of Our Most Contested Right* (Beacon Press 2010);
- *Cybertraps for the Young* (NTI Upstream 2011); and most recently,
- *Cybertraps for Educators* (Mathom Press 2015).

I have also written numerous magazine and newspaper articles on a wide variety of topics, including constitutional rights (particularly freedom of speech), privacy online and in the workplace, the impact of technology on our rights and liberties, and the separation of church and state.

On August 23, 2006, I had the honor of appearing on "The Daily Show with Jon Stewart" to discuss *The Decency Wars: The Campaign to Cleanse American Culture*. I have also appeared as a guest on a variety of other national television programs, including ABC's "Good Morning America Weekend," NBC's "Weekend Today," ABC's "Nightline," CBS's "60 Minutes," and assorted BBC documentaries. In addition to those televised appearances, I have been interviewed by numerous radio shows, magazines, and newspapers around the world on topics relating to my books.

Over the last fifteen years, I have frequently been invited to lecture before college, university, and professional audiences on topics related to my book, including Internet technology, workplace and personal privacy, computer forensics, free speech, and censorship.

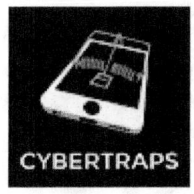

www.ingramcontent.com/pod-product-compliance
Lightning Source LLC
Chambersburg PA
CBHW060245290526
45789CB00001B/201